D1571622

EXERCISES IN DENTAL RADIOLOGY

VOLUME 4

BASIC PRINCIPLES OF ORAL RADIOGRAPHY

MYRON J. KASLE, D.D.S., M.S.D.

Professor and Chairman, Department of Dental Radiology
Indiana University School of Dentistry, Indianapolis,
Indiana

ROBERT P. LANGLAIS, B.A., D.D.S., M.S.

Associate Professor and Director, Graduate Program in
Dental Diagnostic Science, Department of Dental
Diagnostic Science, University of Texas Health Science
Center at San Antonio, San Antonio, Texas.

1981

W. B. SAUNDERS COMPANY   Philadelphia / London / Toronto / Sydney

W. B. Saunders Company: West Washington Square
Philadelphia, PA 19105

1 St. Anne's Road
Eastbourne, East Sussex BN21 3UN, England

1 Goldthorne Avenue
Toronto, Ontario M8Z 5T9, Canada

9 Waltham Street
Artarmon, N.S.W. 2064, Australia

Library of Congress Cataloging in Publication Data

Kasle, Myron J

Basic principles of oral radiography.

(Exercises in dental radiology; v. 4)

Bibliography: p.

Includes index.

1. Teeth—Radiography—Problems, exercises, etc.
   I. Langlais, Robert P., joint author.   II. Title.
   III. Series. [DNLM: 1. Radiography, Dental—Examination
   questions. WN18 K19b]

RK309.K38   617.6'07572   80–51960

ISBN 0–7216–5291–3

Basic Principles of Oral Radiography   ISBN   0-7216-5291-3

Last digit is the print number: 9   8   7   6   5   4   3   2   1

To Professor Olaf Elmer Langland, D.D.S., M.S., F.A.A.D.R., F.A.C.D.
Soldier, practitioner, educator, author, and friend.

CONTRIBUTORS

MAJOR CONTRIBUTORS ————————————————————————

WILLIAM K. BOTTOMLEY,
D.D.S., M.S.
Professor and Chairman
Department of Oral Diagnosis
Georgetown University School of
  Dentistry

D. LORNE CATENA, D.D.S.,
M.Sc.D., F.R.C.D.(C)
Professor of Radiology
Southern Illinois University
  School of Dentistry

BENJAMIN CIOLA, D.D.S., M.S.D.
Chief of Dental Service
V. A. Hospital
West Haven, Connecticut

FELIX CORDERO, R.D.T.
Department of Dental Diagnostic
  Science
University of Texas Health Science
  Center at San Antonio

GORDON M. FITZGERALD, D.D.S.
Professor Emeritus
Department of Oral Roentgenology
University of California at
  San Francisco

H. CLINE FIXOTT, JR., D.D.S.
Professor Emeritus
Department of Oral Radiology
University of Oregon Health
  Science Center

PETER A. FORTIER, B.S., D.D.S.,
M.A.
Professor
Department of Oral Diagnosis and
  Radiology
Louisiana State University School
  of Dentistry

HERBERT H. FROMMER,
B.A., D.D.S.
Professor and Chairman
Department of Oral Radiology
College of Dentistry
New York University Dental Center

RAMESH K. KUBA, B.D.S., M.S.D.
Associate Professor and Director
Oral Radiology Program
University of Minnesota School of
  Dentistry

OLAF E. LANGLAND, D.D.S.,
M.S., F.A.A.D.R., F.A.C.D.
Professor and Director
Division of Oral Roentgenology
University of Texas Health Science
  Center at San Antonio

v

CONTRIBUTORS

T. PAUL McDAVID, D.D.S., M.S.
U.S. Department of the Navy
Washington, D.C.

KEVIN O'CARROLL, D.D.S.,
M.S.D.
Associate Professor and Director
Division of Oral Radiology
University of Mississippi Medical
    Center Dental School

JOHN W. PREECE, D.D.S., M.S.D.
Professor and Director
School of Allied Health
University of Texas Health Science
    Center at San Antonio

AXEL RUPRECHT, D.D.S., M.Sc.D.,
F.R.C.D.(C)
Professor and Chairman
Department of Diagnosis and
    Oral Radiology
University of Saskatchewan School
    of Dentistry

FRANCIS H. SIPPY, B.S., M.S.
Assistant Professor
Department of Oral Pathology and
    Diagnosis
University of Iowa School of
    Dentistry

CARL J. SMITH, D.D.S., M.S.
Department of Oral Diagnosis
Naval Regional Dental Center
Pearl Harbor, Hawaii

FRED M. SORENSON, D.D.S.
Professor and Chairman
Department of Oral Radiology
School of Dentistry
University of Oregon Health
    Science Center

KAVAS THUNTHY, D.D.S.,
M.S.D., M.A.
Associate Professor
Department of Oral Diagnosis and
    Radiology
Louisiana State University School
    of Dentistry

STUART C. WHITE, D.D.S., Ph.D.
Professor and Chairman
Section of Oral Radiology
School of Dentistry
University of California at
    Los Angeles

COLLABORATORS

COLLABORATORS

JAMES W. FRAZER, B.S., Ph.D.
Radiation Specialist
Department of Dental Diagnostic
  Science
University of Texas Health Science
  Center at San Antonio

W. DOSS McDAVID, B.S., M.A.,
Ph.D.
Assistant Professor
Department of Dental Diagnostic
  Science
University of Texas Health Science
  Center at San Antonio

DALE A. MILES, B.A., D.D.S.
Department of Dental Diagnostic
  Science
University of Texas Health Science
  Center at San Antonio

CHARLES R. MORRIS, D.D.S.,
F.A.C.D.
Professor and Chairman
Department of Dental Diagnostic
  Science
University of Texas Health Science
  Center at San Antonio

JOHN REID, D.D.S., M.Sc.D.,
F.R.C.D.(C)
Professor and Director
Division of Oral Radiology
University of Western Ontario
  School of Dentistry

FOREWORD

Get wisdom, get understanding: forget it not...
PROVERBS 4:5

This most recent title in the four-volume series of textbooks *Exercises in Dental Radiology* is a contribution to dental literature that offers an excellent source of pertinent information presented in a manner that challenges and motivates the reader to get wisdom, get understanding, and forget it not.

The first three volumes, *Intra-Oral Radiographic Interpretation* (Vol. 1), *Advanced Oral Radiographic Interpretation* (Vol. 2), and *Pediatric Radiographic Interpretation* (Vol. 3), present material directly applicable to diagnosis and treatment planning. Each volume includes many radiographic illustrations accompanied by specific data to which a unique question-and-answer format is related.

Basic Principles of Oral Radiography should really take precedence in the learning sequence over the previous volumes, since it lays the foundation of principles and practices on which the routine production of anatomically accurate radiographs displaying maximal interpretive qualities is established.

This book is an excellent introduction to the subject of oral radiography and is primarily designed for teaching programs involving dental students, hygienists, assistants, and technicians. A voluminous amount of material has been condensed, illustrated, simplified, and presented in an orderly and readily understandable manner, and the self-testing and self-learning format further adds to the teaching value of the manual. Instructors in oral radiography should welcome this teaching aid with enthusiasm.

The dental practitioner will also find this to be a handy reference source of specific information from which old knowledge can be reinforced and new knowledge acquired.

The authors of these volumes are to be commended for such a unique and helpful contribution to dental literature.

W. J. UPDEGRAVE, D.D.S.

Director of Dental Radiology, The L. D. Pankey Institute for Advanced Dental Education, Miami, Fla.

Professor Emeritus, Temple University School of Dentistry, Philadelphia, Pa.

PREFACE

Volume 4 in the series *Exercises in Dental Radiology* is designed to increase the reader's knowledge of the basic physical, chemical, and biological principles of oral radiography.

In this volume we have treated each major area in several ways. First, the principles are covered using a fill-in-the-blank format. This allows the reader either to learn while reading or simply to confirm that the subject being discussed has been learned and understood. At the end of each section we have included some sample multiple-choice review questions. These questions are based on the material contained in the parent section or in the reference material listed at the end of this volume. All the questions in this volume were supplied by the many contributors to this endeavor.

Additionally, we and our contributors have provided a number of multiple-choice, true-false, matching, and problem-solving questions at the end of this volume. These are in no particular order other than being grouped by type, as would be found on a typical examination.

In this volume we have deviated slightly from our previous format in that we have included the answers on the same page as the question. We have done this for the convenience of our readers. The answers should be covered up and compared with the readers' answers.

Another deviation in format is the material itself. While the other three volumes cover various aspects of oral radiographic interpretation, this volume covers principles. We think that this material is critical to the effective practice of oral radiography.

Finally, we would like to note that this volume is not meant to be comprehensive or to replace the standard dental radiology textbook. We have selectively highlighted the most important aspects of the principles of oral radiography for the edification of our readers. We have included some illustrations that we think will be helpful, and we hope that this unique package will be interesting and entertaining to our readers.

As we have said before, we think that learning should be fun and we most sincerely hope that you enjoy this volume.

M.K.
R.L.

ACKNOWLEDGMENTS

The authors wish to express their sincere thanks to the following persons, without whose help this publication could not have been possible.

First, we would like to thank Carol Ann Steinmetz, Rebecca Cox, Carol Rios, Gwen Haggard, Pat Brownlow, and Stella Schwab for their efforts in typing the manuscript. We also wish to thank Mr. Ray E. Aldrete, Coordinator of Photographic Services at the University of Texas Health Science Center at San Antonio, and Mr. Robert E. Jones, Supervisor of the Technical Illustrations Division, as well as Sheila Palmer and Nancy Reid of the Art Department of the University of Texas Health Science Center at San Antonio, who all did a masterful job of producing excellent quality sketches and diagrams from our original scribblings. We are very thankful to our major contributors. It was their input that provided a broad scope of representative examination material. We are especially grateful to Dr. Olaf Langland, whose unselfish commitment to the advancement of dental knowledge provided us with several unique and outstanding sections as well as a wealth of other material. We are most grateful to our collaborators, whose application of their expertise to this volume has been an enlightening experience. We would like to thank Charles R. Morris, whose encouragement was the single most important contributing factor in the completion of this manuscript.

The authors wish to thank the Eastman Kodak Company, Rochester, New York; the Rinn Corporation, Elgin, Illinois; and Charles C Thomas, Publisher, Springfield, Illinois, along with Olaf E. Langland and Francis H. Sippy for the material that they kindly allowed us to reproduce.

The authors would especially like to thank W. Doss McDavid, whose meticulous in-depth review of the manuscript was most appreciated. As a result of his critique, several areas were revised extensively. His many additions to and deletions of our material have greatly enhanced the quality of this text, for which we are very grateful.

Finally, we must acknowledge the continued support and understanding of our wives, Judy and Denyse.

CONTENTS

SECTION 1

MATTER: THE
STRUCTURE OF THE ATOM

Matter is made of particles that are too minute to be visible to the naked eye. We can see matter because it occupies (1) _____ .

1. space

The person who first postulated that the atom looks like a small solar system was (2) _____ .

2. Bohr

In looking at Figure 1–1 you will note that an atom is made up of a (3) _____ and orbiting (4) _____ . The (5) _____ is heavier than the orbiting (6) _____ .

3. nucleus
4. electrons
5. nucleus
6. electrons

The nucleus contains particles called (7) _____ and (8) _____ . The other particles found in the atom are (9) _____ .

7. protons
8. neutrons
9. electrons

Protons have a (10) _____ electrical charge, where-as neutrons have (11) _____ electrical charge.

10. positive
11. no

Electrons have a (12) _____ electrical charge.

12. negative

An atom normally contains equal numbers of (13)_____ and (14) _____ . This condition thus leaves the atom electrically (15) _____ .

13. protons
14. electrons
15. neutral

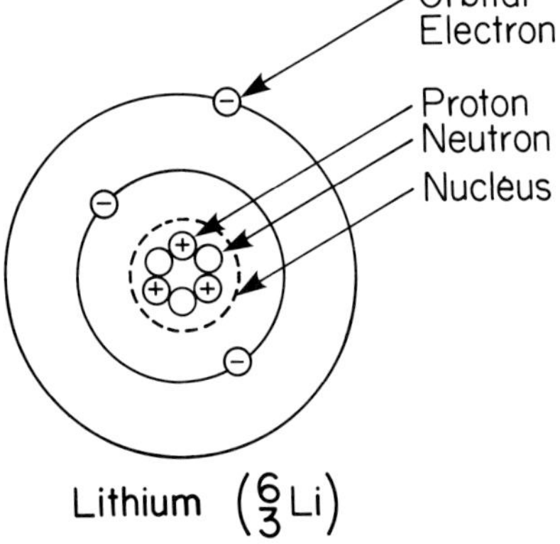

Orbital Electron

Proton
Neutron

Nucleus

Lithium $\left(^{6}_{3}Li\right)$

FIGURE 1–1. Atomic structure.

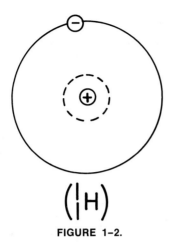

FIGURE 1-2.

Electrons are maintained in their orbits because of electrical attraction to the (16) _____.

16. nucleus

Generally, (17) _____ and (18) _____ are
found in the nucleus of the atom. Because of this they are
called (19) _____. The number of nucleons in an
atom is called the (20) _____, and the sym-
bol used for it is (21) _____. It is often referred to as the
superscript.

17. protons
18. neutrons
19. nucleons
20. mass number
21. A

The number of protons in the nucleus is known as the (22)
_____, and its symbol is (23) _____. It is referred
to as the subscript.

22. atomic number
23. Z

Figure 1-2 illustrates an atomic model of (24) _____.

24. hydrogen

Figure 1-3 illustrates an atomic model of (25)_____.

25. oxygen

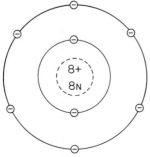

FIGURE 1-3.

The atom in Figure 1–2 has (26) _____ proton(s) and (27) _____ electron(s), whereas the atom in Figure 1–3 has (28) _____ proton(s), (29) _____ neutron(s), and (30)_____ electron(s).

26. 1
27. 1
28. 8
29. 8
30. 8

Electrons surround the (31)_____ in regions called (32) _____.

31. nucleus
32. shells

These (33) _____ are lettered from (34) _____ to _____. The (35) _____ shell is located closest to the nucleus.

33. shells
34. K, Q
35. K

After viewing the illustration in Figure 1–4, identify the parts indicated by numbers 36 to 40: (36) _____, (37) _____, (38) _____, (39) _____, and (40)_____ _____.

36. nucleus
37. K shell
38. L shell
39. electron
40. area where protons
     and neutrons are
     located

IONIZATION

Now that we know what an atom is (you probably knew what it was before we refreshed your memory), let's find out about ionization.

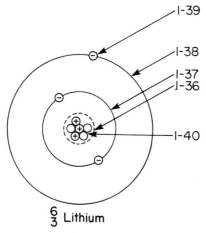

$^6_3$ Lithium

FIGURE 1–4.

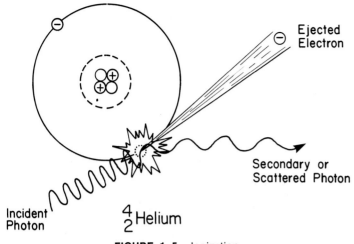

Incident Photon

$^4_2$ Helium

FIGURE 1-5. Ionization.

When an orbiting electron is ejected from its (41)_____ _____ out of the atom, (42) _____ of that atom takes place. This phenomenon is illustrated in Figure 1-5.

41. **shell**
42. **ionization**

The incident photon collides with the orbital electron of the atom being struck. The incident photon gives up some of its energy to the orbital electron with which it collides and ejects the electron from the atom. Once this happens, the atom has become ionized. This means that the electrically neutral atom has been changed into two ions. The first ion is the remainder of the atom that becomes positively charged, and the second, much smaller ion is the ejected electron, which is negatively charged. These ions will react with other ions until new electrically stable (neutral) atoms are formed. Meanwhile, if the incident photon does not give up all of its energy to the electron, it will change direction and continue to react with other atomic particles, such as orbital electrons.

EXCITATION

When an orbiting electron is moved from its usual position in the atom to an orbit farther from the nucleus within the atom, we say that (43) _____ has taken place. So, we see that an atom is affected by (44)_____ and (45) _____.

43. **excitation**
44. **ionization**
45. **excitation**

Atoms that contain the same number of protons but a different number of neutrons in their nuclei are called (46) _____ _____ of the same element.

46. **isotopes**

5

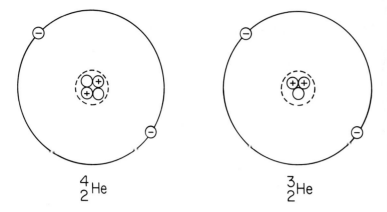

Isotopes of Helium

FIGURE 1-6.

Atoms that have the same mass number but different atomic numbers are known as (47) _____.

47. **isobars**

Sample Examination Questions

1. An atom is said to be neutral when:

   A. It is ionized.
   B. There are more electrons than protons.
   C. The net number of positive charges of the nucleus equals the number of negative charges of the orbital electrons.
   D. It has a positive charge.

2. The electrons that revolve around the nucleus:

   A. Have a positive charge.
   B. Have no charge, either positive or negative.
   C. Have a negative charge.
   D. Can be either positive or negative.

3. Ionization occurs:

   A. When atoms lose electrons; they become deficient in negative charges and, therefore, behave as positively charged atoms.
   B. When atoms gain electrons; they become positively charged.
   C. When an atom loses its nucleus.
   D. Only when a K-orbit electron is ejected and replaced by an L-orbit electron.

4. X rays interact with matter to produce:

   A. Ionization and desiccation.
   B. Ionization and excitation.
   C. Desiccation and excitation.
   D. Ionization and replication.

5. Which electron has the greatest binding energy to the nucleus?

   A. J-shell electron.
   B. K-shell electron.
   C. L-shell electron.
   D. Q-shell electron.

1. C

2. C

3. A

4. B

5. B

6. The structure that has a nucleus containing positive protons with surrounding orbits of one or more negative electrons is called:

   A. A molecule.
   B. A neutron.
   C. An atom.
   D. A proton.

6. C

7. Which of the following statements is true?

   A. The K orbit is closest to the nucleus and its binding energy is the lowest.
   B. The M orbit is farther away from the nucleus and its binding energy is greater than the K orbit.
   C. The K orbit has the greatest binding energy.
   D. The M orbit has the greatest binding energy.

7. C

8. Neutrons have:

   A. A negative charge.
   B. A positive charge.
   C. No charge.
   D. A negative charge on top and a positive charge on the bottom.

8. C

9. Isotopes of an element have the same:

   A. Half-life.
   B. A number.
   C. Z number.
   D. N number.

9. C

SECTION 2

THE COMPONENTS AND
FUNCTION OF THE
DENTAL X-RAY MACHINE

THE DENTAL X-RAY TUBE

Refer to Figure 2–1.

The typical x-ray tube consists of a (1) _____ glass housing from which (2) _____ has been removed. Inside this housing are two (3) _____. One is called the (4) _____, and the other is called the (5) _____. The (6) _____ is the negative electrode, and the (7) _____ is the positive (8) _____. The metal that is shaped like a cup and partially surrounds the cathode is (9) _____.

1. **leaded**
2. **air**
3. **electrodes**
4. **cathode**
5. **anode**
6. **cathode**
7. **anode**
8. **electrode**
9. **molybdenum**

The molybdenum cup is sometimes called a (10)_____ cup. In general, the x-ray tube is surrounded by a special (11) _____ and is housed inside a metal structure commonly referred to as the x-ray unit (12)_____ _____.

10. **focusing**

11. **insulating oil**
12. **head**

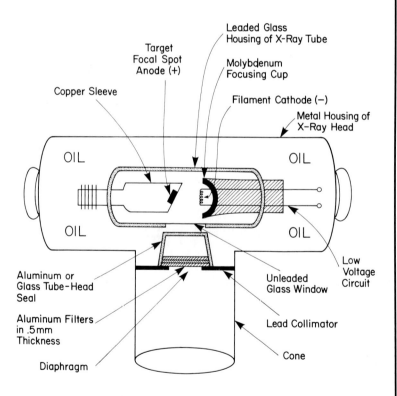

Target
Focal Spot
Anode (+)

Leaded Glass
Housing of X-Ray Tube

Molybdenum
Focusing Cup

Copper Sleeve

Filament Cathode (−)

Metal Housing of
X–Ray Head

OIL

OIL

OIL

OIL

Aluminum or
Glass Tube–Head
Seal

Aluminum Filters
in .5mm
Thickness

Diaphragm

Unleaded
Glass Window

Low
Voltage
Circuit

Lead Collimator

Cone

Schematic Diagram of the Dental X-Ray Head, Tube and Cone

FIGURE 2–1. Construction of an x-ray tube commonly found in the dental x-ray unit.

The cathode is also known as the (13)_____, and it is at this electrode that (14) _____ are produced when a low-voltage electrical current is applied to heat it. The (15) _____ cup is (16) _____ charged like the (17) _____. (18) _____ is a metal that has a high melting point and provides a large number of (19) _____ for (20) _____ emission during heating of the filament.

The (21) _____ is the positively charged electrode. There are two types of anodes: the (22) _____ anode and the (23) _____ anode. Dental x-ray units contain (24) _____ anodes, whereas (25) _____ anodes are commonly found in medical x-ray units. In the typical dental x-ray unit, the anode consists of a block of (26) _____ in which an inlay of (27) _____ has been placed. The inlay of (28) _____ acts as the (29) _____ for (30) _____ that bombard it. These (31) _____ originate in the (32) _____ in the x-ray tube. Copper is a good choice for anode construction because it readily conducts (33) _____ away from the (34) _____ target.

(35) _____ is used as the target material in the construction of the anode for the same reason it is used as the filament in the construction of the (36) _____. What is the reason? (37)_____ _____. This is the main reason, but there are others: Tungsten not only has a (38) _____, but it also has a (39) _____, (40) _____, and (41) _____.

The rotating anode was not introduced until the year (42) _____. During an x-ray exposure, this anode (43) _____ because it is mounted on a shaft that is attached to a small (44) _____. The (45) _____ of the rotating anode during an x-ray exposure prolongs the operating life of the x-ray tube.

Transformers

Transformers are important in an x-ray unit's electrical circuit because they provide the high voltage necessary to produce (46) _____.

13. filament
14. electrons
15. molybdenum
16. negatively
17. cathode
18. tungsten
19. electrons
20. thermionic

21. anode
22. stationary
23. rotating
24. stationary
25. rotating
26. copper
27. tungsten
28. tungsten
29. target
30. electrons
31. electrons
32. cathode
33. heat
34. tungsten

35. tungsten
36. cathode
37. it has a high melting point
38. high melting point
39. high thermal conductivity
40. a high atomic number
41. its cost is relatively low

42. 1936
43. rotates
44. motor
45. movement

46. x rays

Basically, a transformer consists of a piece of (47)_____ with coils of (48) _____ wrapped around it. The copper coils conduct an electric current. The coil that receives the alternating electrical current is called the (49) _____ or (50) _____ coil, and the (51) _____ coil is called the (52) _____ coil. The electrical current that energizes the (53) _____ coil induces another current in the (54) _____ or secondary coil.

47.	iron
48.	copper wire
49.	primary
50.	input
51.	secondary
52.	output
53.	input
54.	output

If there are more wire coils in the secondary than in the primary coils, the transformer is known as a (55) _____ transformer and is used in the high-voltage circuit.

55. step-up

Conversely, if there are more copper wire coils in the primary than in the secondary coils, this is known as a (56) _____ _____ transformer and is used in the low-voltage or filament circuit.

56. step-down

Figure 2–2 is a schematic drawing of typical transformers. Now cover the labels and test how much you remember.

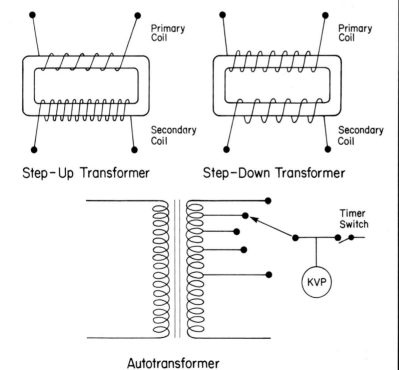

FIGURE 2–2. Typical transformers.

You may have heard the term *autotransformer* (even if you haven't we'll explain what it is). An (57) _____ is a step-down transformer. It controls the voltage applied to the primary coil of the high-voltage transformer. The auto-transformer consists of a single insulated coil of copper wire wound around a core of iron. It is called an (58) _____ _____ because the primary and secondary copper windings are incorporated in a single winding. It forms part of the high-voltage or cathode-anode circuit and is controlled by the kVp selector switch; it is activated by the timer or exposure button.

RECTIFIER/SELF-RECTIFIER.   By using (59) _____ _____, alternating electrical current can be changed into direct electrical current. When an electrical current is (60) _____, the x-ray tube operates more efficiently. The dental x-ray tube is its own rectifier and is commonly called a (61) _____.

KILOVOLTAGE.   Peak kilovoltage probably has the greatest effect on the appearance of the radiographic image. (62) _____ is the maximum potential difference between the cathode and anode electrodes found within the x-ray tube. (63) _____ regulates the penetrating power of the x-ray beam. In dentistry, when one wishes to penetrate structures that are physically thick, such as bone and teeth, the (64) _____ must be increased. Conversely, (65) _____ is decreased if less physically dense materials are to be penetrated.

You will find that an increase in (66) _____ results in a longer scale of image contrast. Contrast becomes greater (short-scale) when a lower (67) _____ is used. X-ray beam (68) _____ is its penetrating ability. Now you know that the penetrating ability of an x-ray beam is dependent on the (69) _____ used and that the (70) _____ of an x-ray beam refers to its penetrating ability.

MILLIAMPERAGE.   Another important factor is milliamperage. This is the amount of electrical (71) _____ that passes through the high-voltage tube circuit. (72) _____ controls the number of (73) _____ produced in the x-ray tube. The (74) _____ of photons of x-ray energy produced is dependent on milliamperage as well as on peak kilovoltage.

57. autotransformer

58. autotransformer

59. rectifiers

60. rectified

61. self-rectifier

62. peak kilovoltage

63. peak kilovoltage

64. peak kilovoltage
65. peak kilovoltage

66. peak kilovoltage

67. peak kilovoltage
68. quality

69. peak kilovoltage
70. quality

71. current
72. milliamperage
73. x-ray photons
74. quantity

Old kVp	50	60	65	70	80	90
50	1	0.5	0.4	0.3	0.19	0.12
60	2.0	1	0.78	0.6	0.37	0.24
65	2.6	1.3	1	0.8	0.48	0.32
70	3.3	1.7	1.3	1	0.62	0.42
80	5.4	2.7	2.1	1.6	1	0.66
90	8.0	4.2	3.2	2.5	1.6	1
	50	60	65	70	80	90

New kVp

FIGURE 2–3. mAs multiplying factors. (From Arthur W. Fuchs, Principles of Radiographic Exposure and Processing, 1958, Courtesy of Charles C Thomas, Publ., Springfield, Illinois.)

In summary, the quantity of x-radiation produced is controlled by (75) _____ and _____, and the penetrating ability of the x rays produced is controlled by (76) _____. We usually see peak kilovoltage abbreviated as (77) _____ and milliamperage as (78) _____. As the time of x-ray exposure is increased, exposure of the radiographic film is increased. Milliamperage and time of exposure are multiplied to arrive at a product called (79) _____. This is usually shown as (80) _____.

75. milliamperage, peak kilovoltage
76. kilovoltage alone
77. kVp
78. mA
79. milliamperage seconds or milliampere seconds
80. mAs or mas

Remember that a new mAs factor is usually required if the kVp is altered. To accomplish this, use Figure 2–3 and multiply the present mAs factor by the factor shown at the intersection of the old and new kVp columns. (To apply this, refer to problems in the Review Section, Part 4, at the end of this volume.)

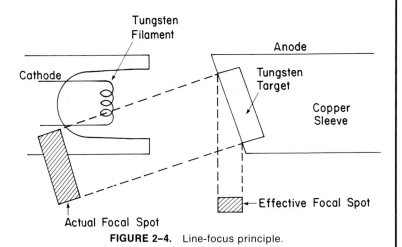

FIGURE 2–4. Line-focus principle.

Line-Focus Principle

In the construction of a dental x-ray tube, the manufacturer must make use of the line-focus principle. In the x-ray tube, the target or focal spot faces the cathode at an angle of approximately (81) _____ (see Figure 2–4).

81. 20°

The effective area of the focal spot is a very small fraction of the focal spot. Radiographic (82) _____ is much better when the x rays are projected from this 20-degree angulation. Later you will see that the smaller the focal spot, the sharper the image.

82. **definition**

Sample Examination Questions

1. The transformer used to heat the filament of the x-ray tube is:

   A. The autotransformer.
   B. The step-up transformer.
   C. The step-down transformer.
   D. The high-tension transformer.

1. C

2. At diagnostic levels, what percent of the electron energy is converted to x-radiation at the anode?

   A. Less than 1%.
   B. 2%.
   C. 10%.
   D. More than 99%.

2. A

3. Approximately 70% of the radiation in an x-ray tube is:

   A. Monochromatic.
   B. Bremsstrahlung.
   C. Characteristic.
   D. Asynchronous.

3. B

4. The step-up transformer is used to:

   A. Step up the current to heat the filament.
   B. Allow the operator to vary the kVp.
   C. Change low-input voltage to high-output voltage with low milliamperage.
   D. None of the above.

4. C

5. The distance from the target to the film is:

   (1) One of the factors that determines the exposure time.
   (2) The only factor that determines the exposure time.
   (3) Increased to use lower kilovoltage.
   (4) Increased to make the beam size small enough to cover the film with as little exposure to the patient as possible.

   A. 1.
   B. 2.
   C. 3.
   D. 1 and 3.
   E. 2 and 4.

5. A

6. The substance that is the most roentgenopaque is:

    A. Leaded glass.
    B. Plastic.
    C. Wood.
    D. Rubber.

6. A

7. If you wished to increase the penetrative quality of x-radiation, how would you change the roentgenographic factors?

    A. Increase the milliamperage (mA).
    B. Increase the kilovoltage (kV).
    C. Increase the mA and the kVp.
    D. Increase the exposure time, the mA, and the (kVp).

7. B

8. Which of the following series shows the correct progression of energy transformation in the production of x-ray photons?

    A. Kinetic energy, electrical energy, and radiation.
    B. Kinetic energy, radiation, and electrical energy.
    C. Electrical energy, kinetic energy, and radiation.
    D. Electrical energy, radiation, and kinetic energy.

8. C

9. Increasing the mA of an x-ray machine increases the:

    (1) Filament temperature.
    (2) Voltage between the anode and the cathode.
    (3) Mean energy of the resultant beam.
    (4) Number of photons generated.
    A. 1 and 2.
    B. 2 and 3.
    C. 1 and 4.
    D. 3 and 4.

9. C

10. X rays are produced when:

    A. The anode is heated above 3000° C.
    B. The filament becomes positively charged.
    C. Positrons strike the anode.
    D. Electrons strike the anode.

10. D

11. Increasing the kVp of an x-ray machine increases the:

    (1) Number of photons generated.
    (2) Mean wavelength of the photons generated.
    (3) Half-value layer of the resultant beam.
    (4) Filament temperature.
A. 1 and 2.
B. 2 and 4.
C. 3 and 4.
D. 1 and 3.

11. D

12. The problem of self-rectified x-ray units is that:

A. A reverse flow of electrons could damage the filament.
B. The tungsten target will melt or pit.
C. The rotor of the rotating anode will not be rotating fast enough.
D. There is not enough penetration to produce useful x rays.
E. B, C, and D.

12. A

13. The dental x-ray beam consists of photons of many different wavelengths, with the shortest wavelength photons determined by:

A. Milliamperage (mA).
B. Kilovoltage peak (kVp).
C. Filtration.
D. Coefficiency of attenuation.

13. B

14. Which of the following statements most adequately describes the radiation produced by high kilovoltage?

A. Short wavelengths of low frequency.
B. Long wavelengths of high frequency.
C. Short wavelengths of high frequency.
D. High penetrating waves of low frequency.

14. C

15. The ideal properties of an anode material include:

    (1) High melting point.
    (2) High atomic number.
    (3) High rate of thermal conductivity.
    (4) High vapor pressure.
    (5) Low vapor pressure.
    (6) Low rate of thermal conductivity.
A. 1, 3, and 5.
B. 2, 3, and 4.
C. 1, 2, 3, and 4.
D. 1, 2, 3, and 5.
E. 1, 2, 5, and 6.

15. D

16. The target material (in the anode) for diagnostic tubes is:

   A. Copper.
   B. Tungsten.
   C. Lead.
   D. Samarium.

16. **B**

17. A dentist decides to change his intraoral exposure technique from 10 mA and 1.5-second exposure to 15 mA and _____ exposure.

   A. 0.38-second.
   B. 1-second.
   C. 2-second.
   D. 6-second.

17. **B**

18. A dentist has been using film Speed D at 65 kVp, 10 mA, and 1-second exposure for a maxillary molar region. His assistant decides to use 15 mA. What will the new exposure time be?

   A. 0.44 second.
   B. 0.66 second.
   C. 0.89 second.
   D. 1.50 seconds.

18. **B**

19. X rays are produced at the:

   A. Filter.
   B. Tip of the cone.
   C. Cathode.
   D. Anode.

19. **D**

20. In a standard dental x-ray unit the *quality* of x-radiation produced during exposure energization is controlled primarily by:

   A. Exposure time.
   B. Kilovoltage (kV).
   C. Milliamperage (mA).
   D. Inherent filtration.

20. **B**

21. Thermionic emission is found at the:

   A. Positive anode.
   B. Negative anode.
   C. Positive cathode.
   D. Negative cathode.

21. **D**

22. The filament circuit in the dental x-ray tube:

    A. Requires a step-up transformer.
    B. Is observed on a voltmeter.
    C. Provides a cloud of electrons when the cathode is heated sufficiently.
    D. Regulates the speed of the electrons.

23. In a standard dental x-ray unit the *quantity* of x-radiation produced during exposure energization is controlled primarily by _____ and _____
_____ .

    A. Exposure time and kilovoltage (kV).
    B. Exposure time and milliamperage (mA).
    C. Exposure time and inherent filtration.
    D. kV and mAs.

24. Increasing the kVp on the x-ray machine will:

    (1) Make caries appear lighter.
    (2) Make caries appear darker.
    (3) Increase the scale of contrast.
    (4) Make everything on the radiograph darker.
    A. 1.
    B. 3.
    C. 2 and 3.
    D. 3 and 4.

25. A .5-second exposure would produce how many "bursts" of x-radiation?

    A. 5.
    B. 15.
    C. 30.
    D. 60.

26. In a step-up transformer the:

    A. Secondary coil has more wire turns than the primary coil.
    B. Primary coil has the same number of wire turns as the secondary coil.
    C. Primary coil has more wire turns than the secondary coil.
    D. None of the above.

27. Some components of the x-ray tube include:

    (1) An anode.
    (2) An aluminum filament.
    (3) Helium.
    (4) Cooling oil.
    (5) A tungsten target.
A. 1 and 5.
B. 3 and 5.
C. 1, 2, and 3.
D. 2, 4, and 5.
E. 2, 3, 4, and 5.

27. A

28. To reduce the amount of heat given off during x-ray production, the source of x-ray energy is surrounded by:

A. Copper.
B. Water.
C. Oil.
D. Lead.
E. Air.

28. C

29. The workload as related to structural shielding design is
a measure of the:

A. Time during which a person to be protected is in the
vicinity of the radiation source.
B. Radiation likely to be produced by an x-ray machine.
C. Time during which the radiation is directed at the
barriers.
D. None of the above.

29. B

30. The number of electrons in a dental x-ray tube is determined by the:

A. Kilovoltage used.
B. Distance between the filament and the target.
C. Step-up transformer.
D. Size of the focusing cup.
E. Low-voltage circuit.

30. E

31. Which of the following is *NOT* related to heat dissipation in an x-ray generating tube?

A. Tube rating.
B. Duty cycle.
C. Copper block.
D. Oil around the tube.
E. Thermionic emission.

31. E

32. In an x-ray generating system, turning the mA control adjusts the:

    A. Filament temperature.
    B. Primary-to-secondary ratio of the step-down transformer.
    C. Primary-to-secondary ratio of the step-up transformer.
    D. Autotransformer.

32. A

33. The instruction booklet accompanying an x-ray machine specifies that the unit should not be energized for more than 17 seconds at the maximum kVp and mA. This is referred to as:

    A. Tube rating.
    B. Duty cycle.
    C. Line-focus principle.
    D. Heat conversion.

33. A

34. The kilovoltage in an x-ray generating system regulates:

    A. The number of electrons produced.
    B. Thermionic emission.
    C. The velocity of electrons travelling from the filament to the target.
    D. The velocity of x-ray photons produced.

34. C

35. The efficiency of x-ray production in an x-ray generating tube (i.e., the percentage of electron kinetic energy converted to x rays) is *directly* related to the:

    A. Z number of the target material.
    B. Operational kVp.
    C. Melting point of the target material.
    D. A and B.
    E. All of the above.

35. D

36. Leakage radiation:

    A. Originates at the focal spot and leaves the tube through the shielding.
    B. Originates at the focal spot and leaves the tube through the unleaded glass window.
    C. Primarily originates in the patient's tissues.
    D. Is significant in image formation.

36. A

SECTION 3

RADIATION: THE
NATURE OF X RAYS

The term *radiation* usually brings to mind some type of force or energy emanating from a body. This energy is associated with either (1) _____ or (2) _____ _____ travelling at high velocities.

1. **electromagnetic waves**
2. **subatomic particles**

Electromagnetic energy is propagated in the form of (3) _____. These waves consist of a (4) _____ field and an (5) _____ field oscillating in perpendicular directions. The energy propagated by (6) _____ _____ is carried in bundles or quanta called (7) _____ _____. Photons carry varying amounts of energy; this energy is proportional to the frequency of the (8) _____ ____.

3. **waves**
4. **magnetic**
5. **electric**
6. **electromagnetic waves**
7. **photons**
8. **radiation**

We deal with a number of electromagnetic radiations every day. Some examples of this are: (9–14) _____, _____ , _____ , _____ _____ , _____ , and _____ .

9. **visible light waves**
10. **heat waves**
11. **radio waves**
12. **gamma rays**
13. **ultraviolet rays**
14. **x rays**

These radiations travel with the speed of light, which is (15) _____ miles per second.

15. $= (3 \times 10^8$ **meters per second)**

Particulate radiation is represented by (16) _____ and (17) _____ particles and (18) _____ and (19) _____ .

16. **alpha**
17. **beta**
18. **protons**
19. **neutrons**

We have learned that electromagnetic energies are propagated by (20) _____ . These waves of oscillating energy are best understood by the illustration in Figure 3–1.

20. **waves**

The measure of one wavelength in Figure 3–1 is that distance between points (21) _____ ; the distance between points (22) _____ is one-half a wavelength. You may therefore say that the distance of the wavelength is from (23) _____ on a single wave train.

21. **A and C**
22. **A and B**

23. **peak to peak**

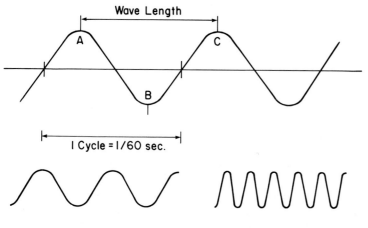

FIGURE 3-1. Electromagnetic waves.

The (24) _____ of the wave is the number of times the wave oscillates in a specific period. The time factor is usually expressed in seconds or fractions of a second. If a 60-cycle current is used, 60 waves will be produced each second.

24. frequency

The speed or (25) _____ of the wave of radiation is the product of the radiation's (26) _____ and (27) _____. The velocities of all electromagnetic radiations are (28) _____ (the same/different). The higher the (29) _____ of an x-ray beam, the greater the photon's (30) _____. Or, the shorter the wavelength of an x-ray beam, the (31) _____ its penetrating power.

25. velocity
26. wavelength
27. frequency
28. the same
29. frequency
30. energy
31. greater

X rays are produced in an x-ray tube by fast-moving (32) _____, which are produced at the (33) _____, striking a target or (34) _____. The speeding (35) _____ slow down because of their interactions with the target (36) _____. A large number of the (37) _____ that enter the target undergo many interactions within the (38) _____ material. The radiation that is produced by this method is called (39) _____. This word is derived from the German term for (40) _____ radiation. This radiation is also referred to as (41) _____. Approximately (42) _____% of the x-ray energy produced in the (43) _____ is in the form of bremsstrahlung. Because it consists of a continuous spectrum containing a variety of wavelengths, it is sometimes referred to as (44) _____ radiation (see Figure 3–2).

32. electrons
33. cathode
34. anode
35. electrons
36. atoms
37. electrons
38. target
39. bremsstrahlung
40. braking
41. bremsrays
42. 70
43. anode

44. "white"

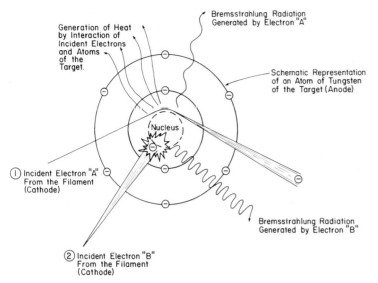

FIGURE 3-2. Generation of heat and heterogeneous bremsstrahlung x-rays at the target.

Now let's talk about characteristic radiation (see Figure 3-3). Electrons are bound in the atom and to their respective shells or (45) _____ by a type of energy called (46) _____. The value of the (47) _____ energy depends on the shell in which the electron is found and the (48) _____ charge. The shell or (49) _____ closest to the nucleus of the atom, the (50) _____ shell, contains the greatest (51) _____ energy. An incoming electron is needed to overcome the binding energy or orbiting target (52) _____.

45. orbits
46. binding energy
47. binding
48. nuclear
49. orbit
50. K
51. binding
52. electrons

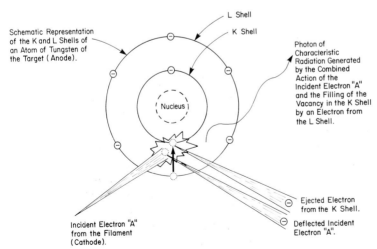

FIGURE 3-3. Generation of characteristic radiation at the target.

If the incoming (53) _____ knock some of the inner (54) _____ out of their (55) _____, electrons from outer shells will "fall down" to fill the vacancies, emitting radiation. The x rays produced by this interaction are known as (56) _____ x rays. As previously mentioned, most x rays are produced by (57) _____ _____. (58) _____ x rays are different for each shell. Characteristic radiation is usually produced only in the (59) _____ and (60) _____ shells of the target atom. For tungsten, K-characteristic radiation is produced at energies greater than 69.5 keV.

53. electrons
54. electrons
55. shells

56. characteristic
57. bremsstrahlung
58. characteristic

59. K
60. L

Sample Examination Questions

1. Electromagnetic radiation wavelengths are measured in:

   A. Kilometers.
   B. Meters.
   C. Angstrom units.
   D. All of the above.

2. To increase the penetrability of the x rays, their wavelengths should be:

   A. Shortened by increasing the kilovoltage.
   B. Lengthened by increasing the kilovoltage.
   C. Shortened by increasing the milliamperage.
   D. Lengthened by increasing the milliamperage.

3. Which of the following are properties of x rays?

   (1) They travel at the speed of light.
   (2) They have a longer wavelength than light.
   (3) They are differentially absorbed by matter.
   (4) They cause chemical changes in matter.
   (5) They precipitate silver from film emulsion.
   A. 1, 2, and 3.
   B. 1, 3, and 4.
   C. 1, 3, 4, and 5.
   D. 2, 3, 4, and 5.
   E. All of the above.

4. Which of the following statements is true?

   A. X rays have wavelengths, frequencies, and velocities.
   B. X rays can be reflected like light.
   C. X rays have mass and carry a positive electric charge.
   D. X rays do not travel in straight lines.

5. Which of the following statements about radiation is true?

   A. General radiation is bremsstrahlung.
   B. Bremsstrahlung is the same as characteristic radiation.
   C. All atoms have the same characteristic radiation.
   D. Characteristic radiation is produced when cathode electrons collide with electrons of the outermost shell.

1.	D
2.	A
3.	C
4.	A
5.	A

6. Which of the following are properties of roentgen rays?

    (1) They are invisible electromagnetic vibrations of high penetrating power.
    (2) They travel at the speed of light.
    (3) They can be focused.
    (4) They are capable of ionizing matter.

A. 1 and 2.
B. 2 and 3.
C. 2 and 4.
D. 1, 2, and 3.
E. 1, 2, and 4.

6. E

7. X rays in the diagnostic range have a wavelength of approximately:

A. 0.01Å
B. 0.10Å
C. 1.00Å
D. 10.00Å

7. B

8. X rays differ from light in that they:

A. Are electromagnetic radiation.
B. Have more energy.
C. Have a greater wavelength.
D. Are usually monochromatic.

8. B

9. Which of the following statements most adequately describes the radiation produced by high kilovoltages?

A. Short wavelengths of low frequency.
B. Long wavelengths of high frequency.
C. Short wavelengths of high frequency.
D. High penetrating waves of low frequency.

9. C

10. To increase the penetrability of the x rays, their wavelengths should be:

A. Shortened by increasing the kVp.
B. Shortened by decreasing the kVp.
C. Lengthened by increasing the kVp.
D. Shortened by increasing the mA.
E. Lengthened by increasing the mA.

10. A

11. Which of the following statements about radiation is true?

    A. Electromagnetic radiation is the propagation of wavelike energy.
    B. Light waves are electromagnetic radiation.
    C. Radio waves are electromagnetic radiation.
    D. Λ and C.
    E. All of the above.

11. **E**

12. Select the correct statement.

    A. X rays cannot be focused to a point.
    B. X rays can be focused to a point.
    C. X rays cannot increase the electrical conductivity of a gas.
    D. X rays do not always travel in a straight line.

12. **A**

13. Secondary radiation is:

    A. Less when kVp is increased.
    B. Most detrimental to the patient.
    C. Less deeply penetrating than primary radiation.
    D. Proportional to the square of the distance the operator stands from the patient.

13. **C**

14. The x-ray beam is:

    A. A continuous beam of radiation.
    B. A convergent beam.
    C. A continuous divergent beam.
    D. A pulsating divergent beam.

14. **D**

15. X rays are used in dentistry because:

    A. They are affected by electric and magnetic fields.
    B. They travel at the speed of light.
    C. They penetrate opaque objects.
    D. They are not differentially absorbed by matter.
    E. They can be focused down to a small area.

15. **C**

16. Which of the following statements is *NOT* correct?

    A. X rays can penetrate opaque matter.
    B. X rays are differentially absorbed by matter.
    C. X rays cannot ionize gases.
    D. X rays affect photographic film emulsion in a manner similar to the action of light.

16. **C**

17. X-radiation:

    (1) Is absorbed by the tissues.
    (2) Scatters.
    (3) Passes through the patient.
    (4) Imparts some or all of its energy to any material through which it passes.

A. 1 and 2.
B. 2 and 3.
C. 2 and 4.
D. 1, 3, and 4.
E. All of the above.

17. E

18. X rays belong to that large group of radiations known as:

A. Particulate radiations.
B. Hygroscopic radiations.
C. Alpha radiations.
D. Corpuscular radiations.
E. Electromagnetic radiations.

18. E

19. The number of oscillations or waves passing a point per second is known as the:

A. Heat capacity of an x ray.
B. Melting coefficient of an x ray.
C. Tube capacity of an x ray.
D. Frequency of an x ray.

19. D

20. Examples of particulate radiation energy include:

    (1) Radar.
    (2) X rays.
    (3) Protons.
    (4) Neutrons.
    (5) Beta rays.

A. 2 and 4.
B. 1, 3, and 4.
C. 1, 4, and 5.
D. 2, 3, and 4.
E. 3, 4, and 5.

20. E

21. Examples of nonparticulate radiation energy include:

    (1) X ray.
    (2) Electron.
    (3) Gamma ray.
    (4) Beta ray.
    (5) Magnetic.

A. 1 and 3.
B. 2 and 4.
C. 1, 2, and 3.
D. 1, 3, 4, and 5.
E. None of the above.

21. A

22. The mean penetrability of an x-ray beam is *NOT* related to which of the following?

A. kVp.
B. Filtration.
C. Wavelength.
D. Frequency.
E. mA.

22. E

23. Increased quantum energy of electromagnetic radiation is associated with increased:

A. LET.
B. Velocity.
C. Frequency.
D. Wavelength.

23. C

SECTION 4

THE INTERACTION OF
X-RADIATION WITH MATTER

When x rays come in contact with various materials, they cause a variety of effects. We have seen the make-up of atoms so we can now better understand the various reactions that take place when x-ray energy passes through them.

X rays have certain properties that make them unique. They are (1) _____ and very (2) _____. Since they are (3) _____ in electrical charge, they (4) _____ be affected by a magnetic field.

1. invisible
2. penetrating
3. neutral
4. cannot

X rays (5) _____ be focused to a point. However, they do affect (6) _____ film, leaving an image on it.

5. cannot
6. photographic

X rays also have the ability to produce (7) _____ and (8) _____ changes in biologic systems. They produce scatter radiation, which is sometimes called (9) _____ radiation. The ability to cause certain materials to (10) _____ makes x rays useful with intensifying screens.

7. physical
8. chemical
9. secondary
10. fluoresce

Certain events may occur when x-ray photons enter matter (see Figure 4–1): (11) _____ scattering may occur, the (12) _____ effect may take place, (13) _____ production may take place, or the (14) _____ effect may occur with absorption of the incident x-ray photon.

11. unmodified (coherent)
12. Compton
13. pair
14. photoelectric

(15) _____ scattering occurs when an x-ray photon interacts with an orbiting electron in an outer shell. The electron may deflect the (16) _____. The photon is scattered without any change in energy. This action occurs more often with low energy x rays.

15. unmodified
16. x-ray photon

The Compton effect occurs when an incident x-ray photon collides with a weakly attached outer-shell (17) _____. If the incident (18) _____ interacts in this manner, it may eject the electron from its outer (19) _____ and then move in a different path. The ejected electron is called a (20) _____ or (21) _____ electron. The original incident x-ray photon is now (22) _____ in energy and emerges from the atom as a so-called (23) _____ photon. The scattered (24) _____ has a longer wavelength, a lower (25) _____, and (26) _____ energy.

17. electron
18. photon
19. shell
20. Compton
21. recoil
22. reduced
23. scattered
24. photon
25. frequency
26. less

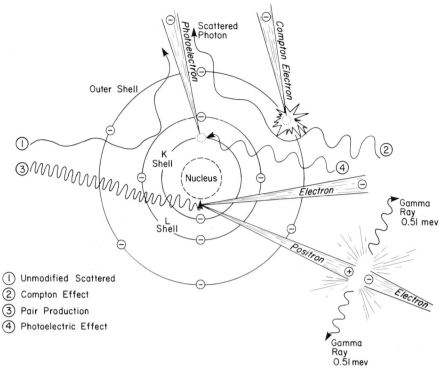

FIGURE 4–1. X-ray interaction with matter.

Pair production occurs when a very energetic incident photon approaches a nucleus. The incident photon is transformed into a (27) _____ of particles: a negative electron and a (28) _____.

27. **pair**
28. **positive electron**

The positive (29) _____ is sometimes called a (30) _____. The (31) _____ interacts with any available (32) _____; this union produces two high-energy photons that move in opposite directions. This reaction is known as the (33) _____ reaction, because the positron and electron give up all of their energies in the production of the two annihilation photons. This interaction does not occur with x rays in the energy range utilized in dentistry.

29. **electron**
30. **positron**
31. **positron**
32. **electron**
33. **annihilation**

Let's say that some material is exposed to x-ray photons. If the energy of the incident photon is great enough to eject a K-shell orbiting electron, then the (34) _____ or (35) _____ occurs. The ejected or removed orbiting (36) _____ is now known as a (37) _____. The incident photon gives up all of its energy in its collision with the orbiting electron and imparts kinetic energy to it. The incident photon completely disappears. This is an example of (38) _____ of the incident photon.

34. **photoelectric effect**
35. **photoelectric collision**
36. **electron**
37. **photoelectron**
38. **absorption**

To reduce the intensity of an x-ray beam, we can place a metal (usually aluminum) in the path of that beam. The (39) _____ layer or (40) _____ is the thickness of the metal that attenuates the x-ray beam intensity to half its initial value.

39. **half-value**
40. **HVL**

As x rays travel farther from their point of origin, that is, from the (41) _____, they diverge or spread out to cover a larger surface area. Their intensity (42) _____ as they travel farther from their source. This is called the inverse square law and can be stated as follows: The intensity of radiation at a certain distance from a point source of radiation is inversely proportional to the square of the distance from that radiation source.

41. **focal spot**
42. **lessens**

Sample Examination Questions

1. Bremsstrahlung is:

    A. The primary source of x-ray photons in the dental x-ray tube.
    B. The process by which x-ray energy is released as electrons rearrange themselves in the inner shells of an atom.
    C. Important only in x-ray machines with rotating anodes.
    D. Not important in the kilovoltage range below 69 kVp.

2. Figure 4–2 is a diagrammatic representation of which of the following types of atomic photoenergy interactions with matter?

    A. Thomson (unmodified) scatter.
    B. The photoelectric effect.
    C. Compton scatter.
    D. Pair production.

3. X rays are known as ionizing radiation. Ionization is:

    A. The separation of the nucleus into positive and negative ions.
    B. Produced by photoelectric absorption only.
    C. Produced by the Compton effect and bremsstrahlung only.
    D. Produced by photoelectric absorption and Compton scatter.

1. A

2. B

3. D

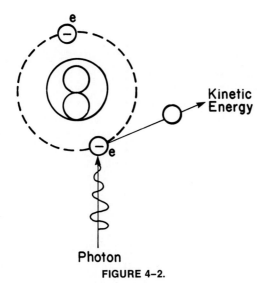

FIGURE 4–2.

4. The interaction in which the entire photon of x-radiation is removed from the beam by atomic interaction is called:

    A. The Thomson effect.
    B. The photoelectric effect.
    C. The Compton effect.
    D. Excitation.

4. B

5. Which of the following statements describes Compton scatter?

    A. The photon uses some of its energy to remove an electron from its orbit and then transfers the remaining energy to the electron in the form of kinetic energy, which is capable of ionizing molecules.
    B. The photon gives up some of its energy in ejecting an orbiting electron and is then deflected with a longer wavelength.
    C. A high-energy photon passes close to a nucleus, releasing an electron and a positron. Some of the energy is used to give kinetic energy to the two particles.
    D. None of the above.

5. B

6. A recoil electron is produced during which of the following interactions?

    A. The photoelectric effect.
    B. The Compton effect.
    C. Pair production.
    D. Photonuclear disintegration.

6. B

7. The interaction of x rays with matter that occurs at diagnostic energy levels and degrades image quality consists mainly of _____ and, to a lesser degree, _____.

    (1) The Compton effect.
    (2) Coherent scatter.
    (3) The photoelectric effect.
    (4) Photonuclear disentegration.
    A. 1 and 2.
    B. 2 and 3.
    C. 3 and 4.
    D. 1 and 4.

7. A

8. Diagnostic radiology is based on which of the following interactions of x rays with matter?

    A. The Compton effect.
    B. Coherent scatter.
    C. The photoelectric effect.
    D. All of the above.

8. D

9. Which of the following are characteristics of photoelectric absorption:

    (1) It depends on atomic number.
    (2) It differentiates between hard and soft tissues.
    (3) It is more likely to occur in inner orbits.
    (4) It does not occur in dental radiography.
    A. 1 and 2.
    B. 2 and 3.
    C. 1, 2, and 4.
    D. 2, 3, and 4.
    E. All of the above.

9. A

10. The predominant mechanism of x-ray interaction with matter in the dental clinical–diagnostic range is:

    A. Thomson (unmodified) scatter.
    B. The photoelectric effect.
    C. Compton scatter.
    D. Pair production.

10. B

11. Dense tissues:

    A. Permit the passage of x rays and are called radiolucent.
    B. Resist the passage of x rays and are called radiolucent.
    C. Resist the passage of x rays and are called radiopaque.
    D. Permit the passage of x rays and are called radiopaque.
    E. None of the above.

11. C

12. Radiopaque tissues:

    A. Absorb little of the x rays.
    B. Absorb x rays more fully.
    C. Are hollow regions.
    D. Are cysts, granulomas, or abscesses.
    E. None of the above.

12. B

13. The extent of absorption of an x-ray beam depends upon the:

    (1) Mean energy of the beam.
    (2) Density of the absorber.
    (3) Thickness of the absorber.
    (4) Speed of the film.

  A. 1 and 2.
  B. 1 and 3
  C. 2 and 3.
  D. 1, 2, and 3.
  E. All of the above.

13. **D**

14. Which of the following statements is true regarding characteristic radiation?

  A. It is produced by the interaction of cathode electrons with target nuclei.
  B. It is produced by the interaction of cathode electrons with target electrons.
  C. It is the major component of the x-ray beam used in dental diagnostic radiology (more than 50%).
  D. A and B.
  E. All of the above.

14. **B**

SECTION 5

FILTRATION AND
COLLIMATION OF THE BEAM

FILTRATION

As the beam travels through the window in the x-ray tube, it is first (1) _____ .

Approximately (2) _____% of the beam consists of bremsrays, and these are not all of the same energy. Some have a short wavelength and a high frequency and are very penetrating; they are therefore useful diagnostically. Other bremsrays have a longer wavelength and are (3) _____ useful diagnostically. Additionally, at energies of 70 kVp and greater, some (4) _____ x rays are produced. Because of the variety of wavelengths in the beam it is called a (5) _____ beam. The low-energy x rays within the beam are not useful diagnostically and are absorbed by the (6) _____ tissues of the patient. This (7) _____ the dose to the patient and provides (8) _____ diagnostic information. Therefore, these nonpenetrating soft x rays should be removed or filtered out of the beam, leaving only the shorter wavelength components. This is accomplished by (9) _____ disks and is called (10) _____ filtration. Added filtration is measured in increments of (11) _____ up to 2.5 mm for most dental machines. The oil, the leaded glass envelope of the x-ray tube, and the leaded glass or aluminum seal are used for (12) _____ filtration. (13) _____ refers to the sum of inherent and added filtrations and is usually expressed in equivalent thicknesses of (14)_____ _____ (measured in millimeters) (see Figure 5–1).

COLLIMATION

Although dental x-ray machines use the line-focus principle, the x-ray beam cannot be (15) _____ . It is, in fact, (16) _____ , much like a beam of light. If the size of the beam were not controlled or collimated, a greater area of the patient's head would be subjected to radiation than is required to expose the (17) _____ . There are two deleterious effects when too large a beam is used: a greater direct dose of radiation from the (18) _____ beam, and a greater somatic and gonadal dose from (19) _____ _____ or (20) _____ radiation originating in the structures irradiated by the primary beam.

1. filtered

2. 70

3. less

4. characteristic

5. heterogeneous or polychromatic
6. soft
7. increases
8. no

9. aluminum
10. added
11. 0.5 mm

12. inherent
13. total filtration
14. aluminum

15. focused
16. divergent

17. film

18. primary

19. secondary
20. scatter

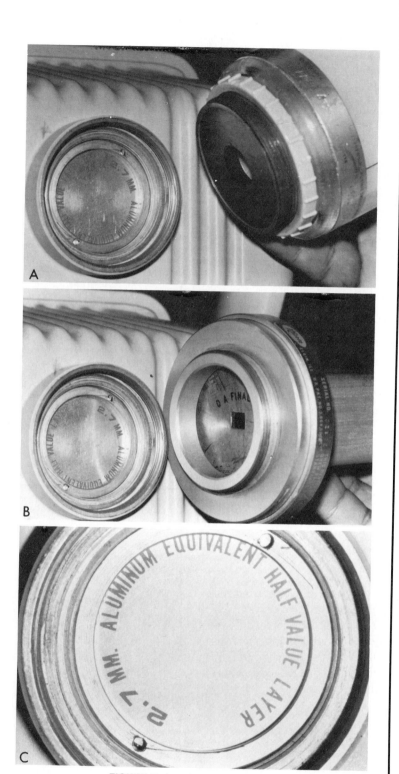

FIGURE 5-1. Aluminum filter.

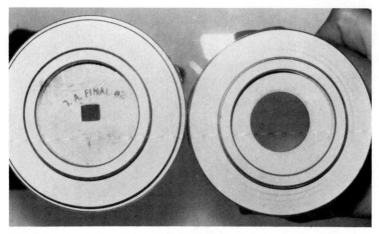

FIGURE 5–2. Collimation. *Left,* Long rectangular cone. *Right,* Short round cone.

Collimation can be accomplished in several ways: (1) A (21) _____ diaphragm at the end of the cone that fits onto the head of the machine can collimate the x rays. The diaphragm is about the size of a quarter for short cones and smaller than a dime for long cones. For a long rectangular cone, the rectangular aperture is smaller than a dime. (2) As the x rays emerge from the diaphragm, they continue to diverge. If they are not kept within the cone, they will be a source of (22) _____ radiation to the patient. By simply lining or impregnating the plastic cone with (23) _____, the x rays can be contained. (3) If a round cone is used, the beam can be further collimated by a (24) _____ collimating and positioning device. The beam, therefore, that has the greatest degree of collimation will result in the smallest dose of radiation to the patient.

21. **lead**

22. **unnecessary**

23. **lead**

24. **rectangular**

Take a look at Figure 5–3. A bite-wing film was placed intraorally on the right side of a dried specimen. An extraoral film was placed on the opposite side of the skull to record the exit dose. The upper bite-wing was taken with the long rectangular cone, and the lower bite-wing with the short round, open cone. Figure A shows the exit dose on the right side, whereas Figure B shows the exit dose on the left side.

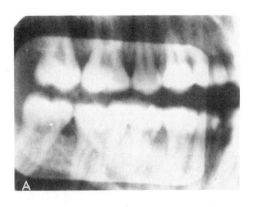

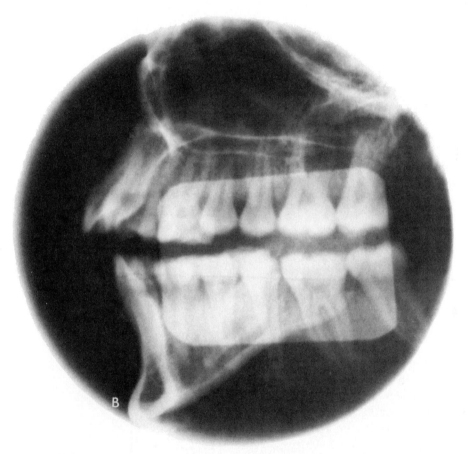

FIGURE 5–3. Exit field, actual size. *A*, Long rectangular cone. *B*, Short cone.

Sample Examination Questions

1. *Collimation* of a beam refers to the:

   A. Selective removal of soft radiation from the beam.
   B. Selective removal of hard radiation from the beam.
   C. Reduction of the beam diameter.
   D. Process of reducing the beam intensity by 50%.

2. Filtration is used in dental x-ray machines to remove:

   A. Scatter radiation.
   B. High-energy photons.
   C. Long-wavelength photons.
   D. Low-energy electrons.

3. The recommended size of the beam at the tip of the cone is:

   A. 2.75 inches.
   B. 3.50 inches.
   C. 4.00 inches.
   D. 5.00 inches.

4. X-ray filters are usually made of:

   A. Copper.
   B. Lead.
   C. Aluminum.
   D. Stainless steel.

5. Collimators are usually made of:

   A. Copper.
   B. Lead.
   C. Aluminum.
   D. Stainless steel.

6. Dental x-ray machines that use more than 70 kVp are required to have a total filtration of at least:

   A. 0.5 mm of aluminum.
   B. 1.5 mm of aluminum.
   C. 2.0 mm of aluminum.
   D. 2.5 mm of aluminum.

1.	C
2.	C
3.	A
4.	C
5.	B
6.	D

7. Collimation is a means of:

    (1) Removing the soft radiations from the x-ray beam and thus reducing the skin dose to the patient.
    (2) Reducing the size of the beam to the patient.
    (3) Increasing the penetration of the x rays.
    (4) Reducing the exit dose from the patient.

    A. 1 and 2.
    B. 1 and 3.
    C. 1 and 4.
    D. 2 and 3.
    E. 2 and 4.

7. E

8. The HVL is the amount of:

    A. Lead necessary to reduce the radiation to zero.
    B. Copper in the target needed to conduct away the heat.
    C. Absorber necessary to attenuate the x-ray beam by one-half and is used to measure the quality of the beam.
    D. Opening in the lead diaphragm needed to collimate the beam to its proper size.
    E. All of the above.

8. C

9. A lead diaphragm is used in dental x-ray machines to:

    A. Prevent Compton scatter.
    B. Limit beam size.
    C. Remove low-energy radiation.
    D. Increase the photoelectric effect.

9. B

10. Proper filtration and collimation of the beam by using a lead diaphragm will:

    A. Reduce scattered radiation fog.
    B. Increase scattered radiation fog.
    C. Not affect scattered radiation fog.
    D. Not absorb divergent secondary rays.
    E. B and D.

10. A

11. The benefits of x-ray beam collimation include:

    (1) Increasing the mean energy of the beam.
    (2) Restriction of the beam size.
    (3) Decreased patient dose.
    (4) Increased quality of the resultant image.

    A. 1 and 2.
    B. 3 and 4.
    C. 1, 2, and 3.
    D. 2, 3, and 4.

11. D

12. Which of the following are characteristics of the central ray of the x-ray beam?

    (1) It is the most concentrated part of the x-radiation beam.
    (2) It is the most direct line of radiation.
    (3) It registers an image with a minimum of distortion.
    (4) If used alone, the fogging action of secondary radiation will be minimized.

A. 1 and 2.
B. 1, 2, and 3.
C. 1, 2, and 4.
D. 2, 3, and 4.
E. All of the above.

12. E

13. Which of the following is true regarding the collimator?

A. It is an aluminum disk with an aperture in the center.
B. It has a smaller aperture for a long cone than a short cone.
C. It removes soft radiation.
D. A and B.
E. All of the above.

13. B

SECTION 6

X-RADIATION MEASUREMENTS

In measuring x-ray output, we universally think in terms of (1) _____ units. This unit of measurement is named after the discoverer of x rays, Wilhelm Conrad (2) _____. The symbol used to signify a (3) _____ measurement is (4) _____.

1. roentgen
2. Roentgen
3. roentgen
4. R

The roentgen is a special unit of (5) _____. Exposure is "the sum of the electrical charges on all of the ions of one sign produced in air when all electrons liberated by photons in a volume of air are completely stopped in air, divided by the mass of air in the volume element" (from National Council on Radiation Protection and Measurements Report No. 35). The roentgen is the exposure required to produce (in air) 2.58×10^{-4} coulombs of ions of either sign per kilogram of air.

5. exposure

Well, if that isn't bad enough, try a rad. Rad is an acronym for (6) _____. It is a unit of absorbed dose, a quantity that describes the amount of energy absorbed per unit mass of any irradiated material. A rad is equal to (7) _____ ergs per gram. When dealing with diagnostic x-ray energies, one R or (8) _____ is approximately equal to one (9) _____ of absorbed dose in (10) _____.

6. radiation absorbed dose
7. 100
8. roentgen
9. rad
10. soft tissue

Now that we know what an R and a rad are in x-ray measurement units, what is a rem? Rem is an acronym for (11) _____. It is the special unit of (12) _____, a quantity used for radiation protection purposes. It expresses, on a common scale for all radiations, the irradiation incurred by exposed persons. Rem is defined as the product of absorbed dose (in rads) and certain modifying factors. The most important of these factors is the (13) _____, which takes into account the fact that different kinds of radiation produce varying amounts of biologic damage. Thus, the dose equivalent in rems is equal to the absorbed dose in rads multiplied by the quality factor. Since the quality factor for x rays is 1, the dose equivalent is equal to the absorbed dose for this kind of radiation.

11. roentgen equivalent mammal
12. dose equivalent
13. quality factor (QF)

MEASUREMENT OF OUTPUT AND HALF-VALUE LAYER

The output of your x-ray equipment may vary as a result of (14) _____, (15) _____, or (16) _____, as well as other causes. The output can be checked using an inexpensive (17) _____ (See Figure 6–1).

14. failure of electronic components
15. removal of a required filter
16. drift from calibration values
17. pocket dosimeter

A pocket dosimeter resembles a pen in size and shape. It contains a simple optical system that permits the user to (18) _____ an internally mounted (19) _____, which serves as the radiation (20) _____. The dosimeter requires a device called the (21) _____. Prior to each use, the dosimeter is (22) _____. This causes the quartz fiber or radiation indicator to be electrostatically (23) _____ by the U-shaped frame upon which it is mounted. The repulsion occurs because both the quartz fiber and the frame receive a (24) _____ charge. When the fiber and frame are fully charged, the hairline image moves to the (25) _____ position.

18. view
19. quartz fiber
20. indicator
21. charger
22. charged (with the charger)
23. repelled

24. positive
25. 0

As you look through the small lens on the end of the dosimeter, a glass disk with calibrated graduations from (26) _____ to (27) _____ may be seen.

26. 0
27. 200 mR (mR = milli-roentgen; 1R = 1000 mR)

When the dosimeter is exposed to ionizing radiation (x rays), the x rays penetrate the sensitive chamber of the dosimeter. This sensitive chamber contains air, and when x rays enter the chamber, the air is (28) _____ to some degree. That is to say, neutral atoms of air are broken down into (29) _____ and (30) _____ ions.

28. ionized
29. positive
30. negative

The wall of the chamber is negatively charged, and the fiber and frame are (31) _____ charged. The positive and negative (32) _____ of air are attracted to to the positively charged fiber and frame and the (33) _____ _____ charged chamber wall. Each time a (34) _____ ion of air combines with the positively charged fiber and frame and a positive ion of air combines with the (35) _____ charged chamber wall, the chamber loses some of its (36)_____.

31. positively
32. ions
33. negatively

34. negative

35. negatively
36. electrical charge

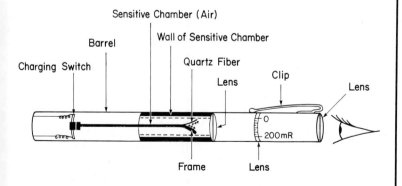

Pocket Dosimeter (Fully Charged)
FIGURE 6–1.

As a result, the positively charged fiber is not as strongly attracted to the negatively charged chamber wall or as strongly repelled by the frame. Thus, the fiber moves from the 0 position on the scale by an amount equal to the radiation exposure received by the (37) _____; this is measured in (38) _____.

Wearing a (39) _____ is a method commonly used to measure the dose an occupationally exposed person may have received. The use of the film badge is based on the fact that film is sensitive to x-radiation; the badge serves as a cumulative record of x-ray exposure during a given period, usually a month. To obtain a film badge one usually subscribes to a film-badge monitoring service. A list of companies that provide this service may be found in *A Textbook of Dental Radiography* by O. E. Langland and F. H. Sippy (Springfield, Ill.: Charles C Thomas, 1975).

Another important type of personnel monitor uses the principle of (40) _____. With this type of dosimetry, a small crystal of a suitable material, such as (41) _____, is used as a dosimeter. When an irradiated crystal of such material is heated in a special TLD "reader," it emits light, which is measured and related to the amount of radiation absorbed. TLD crystals are provided in convenient clip-on badges by the monitoring companies. Like film badges, they are collected and read periodically.

To estimate the output of your machine in mR/mAs at 12 inches, consult Table 6–1. To obtain values for 8- or 16-inch cones, apply the inverse square law (q.v.).

TABLE 6–1. MEAN MILLIROENTGENS PER MILLIAMPERE SECOND AT 12 INCHES BY KILOVOLT PEAK AND FILTRATION CATEGORIES FOR DENTAL X-RAY UNITS*

Total filtration (millimeters of Al equivalent)	Kilovolt peak								
	50	55	60	65	70	75	80	85	90
0.5	91.11	96.03	101.44	107.59	114.73	123.10	132.94	144.49	158.00
1.0	58.38	63.32	68.54	74.27	80.75	88.24	96.98	107.20	119.15
1.5	36.61	41.64	46.72	52.09	57.99	64.66	72.35	81.30	91.75
2.0	23.26	28.45	33.45	38.52	43.89	49.81	56.52	64.25	73.27
2.5	15.79	21.19	26.19	31.01	35.92	41.14	46.93	53.52	61.16
3.0	11.65	17.33	22.37	27.02	31.52	36.12	41.04	46.55	52.88
3.5	8.30	14.32	19.47	24.01	28.17	32.19	36.32	40.80	45.88
4.0	3.19	9.61	14.94	19.43	23.30	26.82	30.21	33.73	37.62
4.5	—	.67	6.24	10.73	14.39	17.46	20.18	22.80	25.56

*From *Population Exposure to X-Rays, US 1964.* US Public Health Service Publication No. 1519. US Public Health Service, Oct. 1966.

Sample Examination Questions

1. The unit for measuring x-ray exposure in air is called the:

   A. Roentgen.
   B. rad.
   C. Roentgenogram.
   D. Radiogram.
   E. Radiograph.

   1. A

2. X-radiation is absorbed by tissues during a diagnostic exposure. The radiation absorbed dose equivalent in man is expressed in rems. Rems are calculated by using:

   A. Roentgens (R) × linear energy transfer (LET).
   B. rads × quality factor (QF).
   C. R × QF.
   D. rads × LET.

   2. B

3. Pocket dosimetry is an example of:

   A. Chemical dosimetry.
   B. Photographic dosimetry.
   C. Luminescent dosimetry.
   D. Biologic dosimetry.
   E. Air-ionization dosimetry.

   3. E

4. Which of the following is *NOT* applicable to thermoluminescent dosimetry?

   A. Ultraviolet light.
   B. Heat.
   C. Trapping centers.
   D. Lithium fluoride.
   E. Measurement of light.

   4. A

5. The quality factor is used in the determination of which of the following radiation units?

   A. R.
   B. rad.
   C. rem.
   D. QF.

   5. C

6. The unit of x-radiation measurement that deals with the absorbed energy per gram of tissue is the:

    A. Roentgen.
    B. rad.
    C. rem.
    D. QF.

6. B

7. The quartz fiber in a pocket dosimeter is:

    (1) Positively charged.
    (2) Negatively charged.
    (3) The indicator.
    (4) Unaffected by ionizing radiation.
    A. 1 and 3.
    B. 2 and 4.
    C. 2 and 3.
    D. 3 and 4.

7. A

8. The sensitive chamber of a pocket dosimeter:

    (1) Contains air.
    (2) Has a negatively charged wall.
    (3) Contains a vacuum.
    (4) Is where ionization occurs.
    A. 1 and 2.
    B. 2 and 3.
    C. 1, 2, and 4.
    D. 2, 3, and 4.

8. C

9. A pocket dosimeter should be _____ before each use.

    A. Checked for x-ray translucency.
    B. Sensitized with a standard radiation exposure.
    C. Loaded in the darkroom.
    D. Charged with the charging unit.

9. D

10. A film badge:

    (1) Is affected by ionizing radiation.
    (2) Is affected by other forms of radiant energy such as heat.
    (3) Should be worn by all occupationally exposed persons.
    (4) Is used to identify x-ray films.
    A. 4.
    B. 1 and 3.
    C. 1, 2, and 3.
    D. 1, 3, and 4.

10. C

THE QUALITY IMAGE: GEOMETRIC FACTORS, DENSITY, AND CONTRAST

Olaf E. Langland

The *image* is a reproduction of various details of the anatomic structures through which the (1) _____ beam has passed. These details are defined by varying degrees of sharpness and shape, depending on the (2) _____ conditions present at the time of exposure. Because of these (3) _____ characteristics, there is a certain amount of unsharpness, magnification, and shape distortion of the radiographic image in all radiographs.

There are three reasons for unsharpness, magnification, and distortion (see Figure 7–1): (1) X rays originate from a definite (4) _____ rather than a (5) _____ source. The area of the source (target) in modern dental x-ray machines varies from (6) _____ mm to (7) _____ mm square, depending on the (8) _____ and (9) _____ of the machine. (2) X rays travel in (10) _____ straight lines as they radiate from the source. This causes (11) _____ _____ of the object. The magnification factor can be minimized by (12) _____ the source-film distance and (13) _____ the object-film distance. (3) The structures of the human jaws have depth as well as length and width. This results in (14) _____

1. **x-ray**

2. **geometric**

3. **geometric**

4. **area**
5. **point**
6. **0.8**
7. **1.5**
8. **mA**
9. **kVp**
10. **diverging**
11. **magnification**
12. **increasing**
13. **decreasing**
14. **unequal**

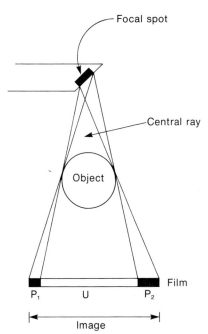

FIGURE 7–1. Reasons for unsharpness, magnification, and distortion in every radiograph. Areas P$_1$ and P$_2$ are zones of image fuzziness called *penumbra*. The area between P$_1$ and P$_2$ is the *umbra* or image of the actual size of the object. Areas P$_1$, U, and P$_2$ together are the magnified image of the object as seen on the film. (Adapted from O. E. Langland and F. H. Sippy, Textbook of Dental Radiology, Revised 1st Edition, 1975, Courtesy of Charles C Thomas Publisher, Springfield, Illinois.)

magnification (shape distortion) of various parts of the anatomy. Those structures at a (15) _____ distance from the film, such as the buccal roots of the maxillary molars and the zygoma, will show increased (16) _____ _____ and (17) _____ in comparison to the structures closer to the film. The same observation can be made at the facial and lingual surfaces of the interproximal bone as well as at the buccal and lingual cusps of the posterior teeth.

15. **greater**

16. **magnification**
17. **unsharpness**

UMBRA AND PENUMBRA

Umbra is the Latin word meaning (18) _____. If a beam of light (visible) is directed at an object placed in front of a screen (recording surface), a shadow of the object will be seen. Shadows with sharply defined margins are called (19) _____. X rays behave much like light rays except that they are (20) _____ and they (21) _____ opaque objects. Like light rays, x rays directed at an object in front of a recording surface (film) will cast a shadow (image) on the surface. Under certain circumstances, the shadow or image will enlarge and its edges will become fuzzy and indistinct. This area of unsharpness or fuzziness is known as the (22) _____.

18. **shadow**

19. **umbras**
20. **invisible**
21. **penetrate**

22. **penumbra**

Before we go on, remember that every radiograph will have a certain degree of unsharpness, magnification, and distortion owing to factors over which you have no control. Additionally, we have introduced the terms *umbra* and *penumbra*. Now we want to discuss those factors you can control to some degree. Since they are not fixed or constant, they should be adjusted in a manner whereby the image will most accurately resemble the object (within the limitations imposed by the variable factors mentioned above).

PRINCIPLES OF ACCURATE IMAGE PROJECTION

1. The x rays should proceed from as small a (23)_____ _____ as conditions allow.

23. **focal spot**

2. The source-object distance should be as (24) _____ _____ as possible.

24. **long**

3. The object-film distance should be as (25) _____ as possible.

25. **short**

4. As far as is practical, the long axis of the (26) _____ _____ should be (27) _____ to the film.

26. object
27. parallel

5. The central ray should be as nearly (28) _____ _____ to the film as possible. This makes it possible to record adjacent anatomic structures in their true (29) _____.

28. perpendicular

29. spatial relation-
     ships

OBJECTIVES OF DENTAL RADIOGRAPHIC PROJECTION TECHNIQUES

1. Increase definition by decreasing geometric unsharpness or size of the penumbra.

Definition is a (30) _____ feature of the film image and refers to the distinctiveness and (31) _____ demarcation of all details of the image. Definition is usually referred to as sharpness or unsharpness of the image. Definition is controlled by (32–37) _____, _____, _____, _____, _____, and _____. Geometric unsharpness is the fuzzy outline caused by penumbra and, as you can see in Figures 7–2 and 7–3, is controlled by (38–40) _____, _____, and

30. qualitative
31. sharp

32. source-object
     distance
33. object-film distance
34. focal spot size
35. film grain size and
     thickness
36. screen grain size
     and thickness

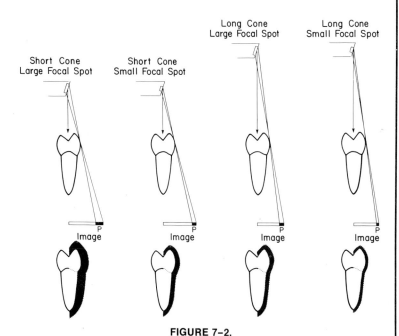

Short Cone Large Focal Spot   Short Cone Small Focal Spot   Long Cone Large Focal Spot   Long Cone Small Focal Spot

Image   Image   Image   Image

FIGURE 7–2.

58

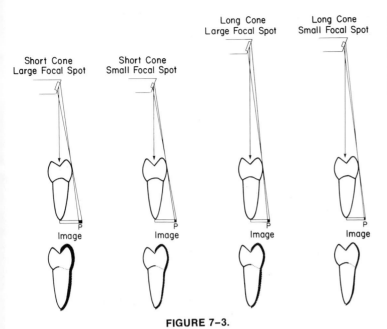

| Short Cone Large Focal Spot | Short Cone Small Focal Spot | Long Cone Large Focal Spot | Long Cone Small Focal Spot |

FIGURE 7–3.

_____. The width of the zone of geometric unsharpness or penumbra can be illustrated by the following formula:

$$P = \frac{FS \times d}{D}$$

where P = Penumbra size (mm)
    FS = Focal spot size
    d = Object-film distance

D = Source-object distance

2. **Decrease magnification of anatomic structures, especially the teeth.**

Magnification is the enlargement of the actual size of the (41) _____ on the radiographic image. As can be seen in Figure 7–4, the degree of enlargement is a function of the (42) _____ and (43) _____ distances. Magnification is minimized by (44) _____ the source-film distance and (45) _____ the object-film distance. The percentage of magnification of an object at any source-film distance (SFD) and object-film distance (OFD) can be readily determined by the following formula:

$$\frac{SFD}{SFD - OFD} - 1 \times 100\% = \text{percentage of magnification}$$

Example: $\frac{17}{17 - 1} - 1 \times 100\% = 6.25\%$

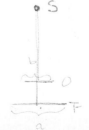

Magnification or Equal Enlargement

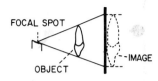

8 inch Focal Film Distance

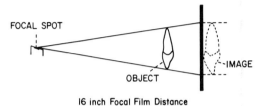

16 inch Focal Film Distance

Comparison of 8 inch and 16 inch Focal Film Distance

FIGURE 7-4. From "New Horizons in Periapical Radiography." Courtesy of the Rinn Corporation, Elgin, Illinois.

The source-film distance divided by the source-object distance is called the (46) _____.

The actual size of the tooth can be calculated by using the following formula (if foreshortening and elongation are not factors):

$$\frac{\text{actual length of tooth}}{\text{length of x-ray image of tooth}} = \frac{\text{source-object distance}}{\text{source-film distance}}$$

$$\text{Example:} \quad \frac{X}{24.5 \text{ mm}} = \frac{16.3}{17.3}$$

$$X = 23.1 \text{ mm}$$

3. **Decrease dimensional distortions of the radiographic image such as elongation, foreshortening, and overlapping of images of anatomic structures (Figure 7–5).**

Dimensional distortion of a radiographic image is a variation of the (47) _____ of an anatomic structure. It results from improper alignment of the film with the (48) _____ and the (49) _____ with the film. Dimensional distortion can be minimized by placing the film (50) _____ to the major planes of the object and

46. **magnification factor**

47. **true size**

48. **object**
49. **radiation beam**
50. **parallel**

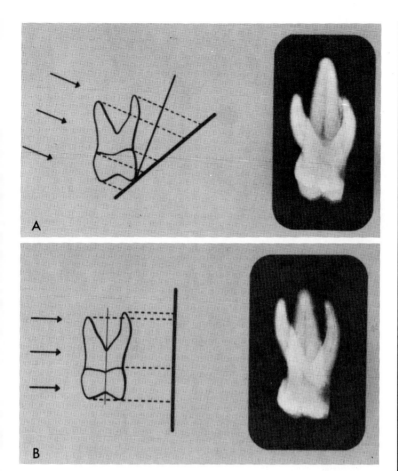

FIGURE 7–5. Dimensional or shape distortion or unequal enlargement. *A,* Bisecting angle in short-cone technique. *B,* Paralleling in extension tube technique. (From Updegrave, W. J.: Simplifying and improving intraoral dental roentgenography. Oral Surg. *12*(6):706, 1959.)

directing the central ray (51) _____ to the major planes of the object and (52) _____. If there is an angle between the film and the object, foreshortening occurs as a result of (53) _____ angulation; elongation is caused by (54) _____ angulation. Overlapping of structures, such as interproximal contacts, is caused by an improper alignment of the (55) _____ and the (56) _____ angulation of the beam. When this occurs, the horizontal angle of the beam is corrected mesially or distally, according to the relationship of the buccal and lingual cusps and the use of the buccal-object rule or Clark's rule (see Section 8).

4. **Increase anatomic accuracy (shape distortion) by recording adjacent anatomic structures in their true spatial relationships (Figure 7–6).**

Anatomic accuracy is achieved when the structures are reproduced on the film in their true (57) _____

51. **perpendicular**
52. **film**

53. **excessive vertical**
54. **insufficient vertical**

55. **film**
56. **horizontal**

57. **spatial relationships**

Anatomical Accuracy

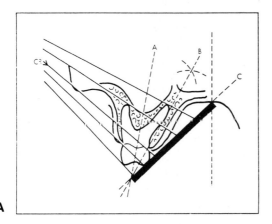

A

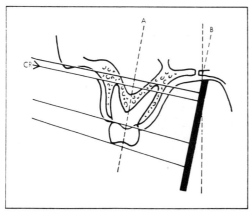

B

FIGURE 7–6. *A,* Bisecting projection technique. In bisecting technique parts of the anatomic structures farther away from the film are projected in an incorrect relationship to parts closer to the film. *B,* Paralleling technique. (From O. E. Langland and F. H. Sippy, Textbook of Dental Radiography, Revised 1st Edition, 1975, Courtesy of Charles C Thomas, Springfield, Illinois.)

_____. Shape distortion interferes with anatomic accuracy because it (58) _____ the resulting radiographic images so that they no longer represent the true (59) _____ of the object being radiographed. The radiographic image is said to have anatomic accuracy when: the labial and lingual cementoenamel junctions of the anterior teeth are (60) _____; the buccal and lingual cusps of the posterior teeth are (61) _____; the contacts of the teeth are (62) _____; the buccal portion of the alveolar crest is (63) _____ over the lingual portion of the alveolar crest; and there is no (64) _____ of the malar process of the zygomatic arch over the roots of the maxillary molars.

58. alters

59. shape

60. superimposed
61. superimposed
62. opened
63. superimposed

64. superimposition

RADIOGRAPHIC IMAGERY: PUTTING IT ALL TOGETHER

The image that has been projected onto the radiographic film must be an image of good diagnostic quality. Proper diagnosis and interpretation of a radiograph depend on the density, contrast, definition, detail, and minimal distortion of the image.

The density of radiographic film is the amount of (65) _____ _____ viewed on the developed film. Very minute clumps of black (66) _____ silver are developed after exposure to ionizing radiation; these minute clumps contribute to the (67) _____ of the film. A typical radiograph, if it has been properly exposed to x rays and properly developed, will normally show areas of different (68) _____. These density differences are commonly regarded as radiographic (69) _____.

The (70) _____ of a radiographic image depends on several factors: the film, the development process, and the make-up of the radiographed object.

(71) _____ can be controlled by the chemical development of radiographic film. (72) _____ and (73) _____ variables of film development, if followed as closely as possible, will result in a film of optimal (74) _____. If enough time is not allowed for proper film development or if the processing solutions are too cold for optimal development, the radiographic image will not be (75) _____ or (76) _____ and will certainly not have proper (77) _____. The reverse is also true; if too much time is given for film development or if the processing solutions are too hot for optimal development, the radiographic image will have too much density and will lack proper (78) _____.

Kilovoltage is adjusted to alter object (79) _____. A short-scale contrast image is produced at (80) _____ kVp ranges; long-scale contrast is produced at high kVp ranges.

The (81) _____ in a radiograph depends on the amount of (82) _____ or (83) _____. Contrast is also involved in (84) _____. If the contrast is poor, it is likely that image (85) _____ will also be poor. A radiograph has good (86) _____ when the images are (87) _____ and easily viewed and when density and contrast are optimal.

To provide a radiographic image with good (88) _____ and (89) _____, we must start with the smallest practical (90) _____ spot in the x-ray generating

65. **blackness**

66. **metallic**

67. **density**

68. **densities**

69. **contrast**

70. **contrast**

71. **contrast**
72. **time**
73. **temperature**

74. **contrast**

75. **clear**
76. **definitive**
77. **contrast**

78. **contrast**

79. **contrast**
80. **low**

81. **detail**
82. **sharpness**
83. **definition**
84. **detail**
85. **detail**
86. **detail**
87. **sharp**

88. **detail**
89. **definition**
90. **focal**

tube. You will lose (91) _____ of the image if there is movement during radiographic exposure. Loss of definition is referred to as (92) _____. Definition of an image is referred to as (93) _____ of an image.

The time needed to produce an adequate image on a radiographic film is also important in reducing the possibility of image (94) _____. Exposures should be made as quickly as possible to reduce image motion (95) _____. If the film, patient, or x-ray generating equipment moves during radiographic exposure, the image produced will probably demonstrate motion (96) _____.

(97) _____ of an image may also be caused by the type of radiographic film used. The faster (98) _____ have larger (99) _____. This processed film will appear more grainy than the (100) _____ films, which contain smaller (101) _____. Images on the faster films appear lacking in (102) _____ and less sharp than the so-called (103) _____ films. You may have heard the term *radiatized film* used for the slower films. Fortunately, the use of faster films has not hindered the clinician in film interpretation and diagnosis. The use of faster films has enabled the dentist to produce radiographs more rapidly, with the benefit of less radiation to the patient. There is a trade-off here. The faster films may not have the fine definition that the slower radiatized films have, but their use is the single most important factor in reducing radiation exposure to the patient in modern dental radiography.

What about the image we view in the radiograph? It has been mentioned that the smaller the target or (104) _____, the better the definition of the radiographic (105) _____. The image is called the (106) _____, and the area at the edge of the image is called the (107) _____. A wide (108) _____ imparts lack of definition to an image, and thus we see an unsharp image. The (109) _____ of an image decreases as the (110) _____ distance increases. Decreasing the object-film distance (111) _____ the size of the (112) _____. What happens to definition or (113) _____? You're right if you said that definition becomes (114) _____.

The latent image is the (115) _____ image in the film (116) _____ that is eventually converted to a

91. **definition**

92. **unsharpness**
93. **sharpness**

94. **unsharpness**

95. **unsharpness**

96. **unsharpness**

97. **unsharpness**
98. **films**
99. **silver grains**
100. **slower**
101. **silver grains**
102. **definition**
103. **slower**

104. **focal spot**
105. **image**
106. **umbra**
107. **penumbra**
108. **penumbra**
109. **penumbra**
110. **focus-film**
111. **decreases**
112. **penumbra**
113. **sharpness**
114. **better**

115. **invisible**
116. **emulsion**

(117) _____ image when chemically developed in the (118) _____.

Radiographic resolution is the ability of a radiograph to record (119) _____. Fine discussions of resolution can be found in Goodwin, Quimby, and Morgan, *Physical Foundations of Radiology,* and in Johns and Cunningham, *The Physics of Radiology* (see References).

117. **visible**
118. **darkroom**

119. **image detail**

Sample Examination Questions

1. Which of the following properties of x rays is the basis for the rules of geometric projection?

   A. X rays travel at the speed of light.
   B. X rays travel in diverging straight lines from a point source.
   C. The course of an x-ray photon can be diverted with an electromagnetic source.
   D. X rays can form a latent image on photographic film.

   1. **B**

2. Regardless of the target-film distance, incorrect horizontal angulation will cause:

   A. Elongation of the x-ray image.
   B. Foreshortening of the x-ray image.
   C. No significant change in the x-ray image.
   D. Overlapping of teeth in the x-ray image.

   2. **D**

3. Figure 7–7 is a diagrammatic representation of an anode inclined at a 20° angle to vertical. This demonstrates the Benson line-focus principle, which is used to:

   A. Increase efficiency of x-ray production.
   B. Serve as an x-ray focusing device.
   C. Produce an effectively smaller focal spot.
   D. Dissipate heat from energy conversion.

   3. **C**

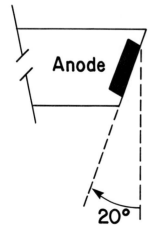 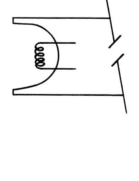

FIGURE 7–7.

4. Figure 7–8 is a diagrammatic representation of x-radiation emanating from the focal spot (FS) of the anode. The sharpness of the image is, in part, controlled by the size of the focal spot. Because radiation is emitted in all directions, the resultant image exposure field shows a central zone of clarity and a peripheral zone of unclarity. This central zone of clarity (CZC) is known as the:

   A. Umbra.
   B. Heel effect.
   C. Penumbra.
   D. Zone of contrast.

4. A

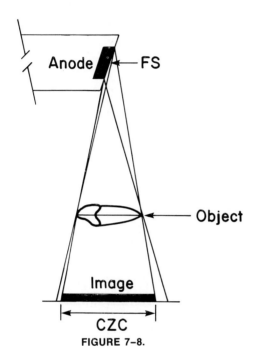

FIGURE 7–8.

5. The size of the x-ray tube focal spot influences radiographic:

   A. Density.
   B. Contrast.
   C. Definition.
   D. Distortion.

5. C

6. Which of the following does *NOT* control magnification of the radiographed object?

   A. Focal spot–film distance.
   B. Alignment of film, objects, and radiation cone.
   C. Object-film distance.
   D. Cathode size.

6. D

7. In the paralleling technique, an increased source-object distance:

   A. Prevents enlargement of the image.
   B. Avoids overlapping.
   C. Prevents shadows.
   D. Causes blurring of the image outline.
   E. None of the above.

7. A

8. Which property of x-radiation must be utilized to control magnification of the radiographic image?

   A. X rays travel in divergent paths from their source.
   B. X rays penetrate opaque objects.
   C. X rays cannot be focused.
   D. X rays cause secondary radiation when they strike the patient's face.

8. A

9. A large focal spot permits:

   (1) More radiation and hence a sharper picture.
   (2) Less radiation and hence a sharper picture.
   (3) Better collimation.
   (4) Poorer definition on the radiograph.
   A. 1.
   B. 3.
   C. 4.
   D. 2 and 3.
   E. 2 and 4.

9. C

10. Minimum magnification and maximum definition are best achieved by what combination of the following?

    (1) Minimum object-film distance (OFD).
    (2) Maximum focal spot–film distance (FFD).
    (3) Maximum OFD.
    (4) Minimum FFD.
    A. 1 and 2.
    B. 1 and 4.
    C. 2 and 3.
    D. 2 and 4.
    E. None of the above.

10. A

11. The advantages of the smallest possible focal spot are:

    (1) Decreased geometric unsharpness.

11. B

     (2)   Decreased filtration.
     (3)   Increased definition.
     (4)   Decreased danger from scatter radiation.
A.   1 and 2.
B.   1 and 3.
C.   2 and 3.
D.   3 and 4.

12.   What are the factors requisite to obtain the least degree of magnification of the roentgenographic image?

     (1)   The smallest possible focal spot size.
     (2)   The recommended amount of total filtration.
     (3)   The longest focal spot–film distance consistent with the roentgenographic technique being used.
     (4)   The shortest practical object-film distance.
A.   1 and 2.
B.   1 and 3.
C.   2 and 3.
D.   3 and 4.

12. D

13.   Factors that contribute to optimal detail sharpness include:

     (1)   A small focal spot area.
     (2)   Increased kilovoltage (kV).
     (3)   A long focal spot–film distance.
     (4)   A short object-film distance.
A.   1 and 2.
B.   1 and 3.
C.   2 and 3.
D.   3 and 4.
E.   1, 3, and 4.
F.   2, 3, and 4.

13. E

14.   The advantages of using an increased cone distance are:

     (1)   Increased contrast.
     (2)   Increased sharpness.
     (3)   Reduced magnification.
     (4)   Reduced shape distortion.
A.   1 and 2.
B.   1 and 3.
C.   2 and 3.
D.   3 and 4.

14. C

15. The density of an intraoral film indicates the:

   A. Degree of darkness.
   B. Difference between dentists.
   C. Speed of the screens.
   D. Kilovoltage used.
   E. None of the above.

16. Which of the following would you do to increase film density?

   (1) Increase the mA.
   (2) Increase the kVp.
   (3) Increase the time.
   (4) Decrease the distance.
   (5) Increase the distance.
   A. 1, 2, and 4.
   B. 1, 2, and 5.
   C. 1, 3, and 4.
   D. 1, 3, and 5.
   E. 1, 2, 3, and 4.

17. Density is a function of:

   A. kVp.
   B. mA.
   C. mAs.
   D. Exposure time.
   E. All of the above.

18. Dental tissues absorb radiation in different amounts because of their varying densities. This differential absorption causes tissue contrast in the processed radiograph. In addition, the film itself has certain properties that dictate contrast, as do the physical factors of the x-ray apparatus. Contrast in the finished radiograph is defined as the:

   A. Varying densities between black and white.
   B. Overall blackening of the film.
   C. Degree of overall grayness of the film.
   D. None of the above.

19. Contrast is primarily a function of:

   A. Kilovoltage.
   B. Kilovoltage and milliamperage.

C. Milliamperage.
D. Kilovoltage, milliamperage, and time.

20. An increase in which of the following factors causes an increase in contrast?

    A. Time of exposure.
    B. Milliamperage.
    C. Kilovoltage.
    D. None of the above.

20. D

21. Increasing the kVp results in:

    A. Low contrast (long-scale contrast).
    B. High contrast (short-scale contrast).
    C. Lighter film density (medium-scale contrast).
    D. None of the above.

21. A

22. How does long-scale contrast affect the interpretive value of a roentgenogram?

    (1) It increases the grades of differences between the roentgenographic densities in the roentgraphic images.
    (2) It increases the detail recorded in the roentgenogram.
    (3) It reduces the interpretive value of the roentgenogram.
    (4) It decreases the detail recorded in the roentgenogram.
    A. 1 and 2.
    B. 1 and 3.
    C. 1 and 4.
    D. 2 and 3.
    E. 2 and 4.
    F. 3 and 4.

22. A

23. Increasing kVp only causes:

    (1) Increased density.
    (2) Decreased density.
    (3) Increased contrast.
    (4) Decreased contrast.
    A. 1 and 3.
    B. 1 and 4.
    C. 2 and 3.
    D. 2 and 4.

23. B

24. Fog affects the contrast of an intraoral film because it:

    A. Decreases film density.
    B. Increases film density.
    C. Produces white specks on the film.
    D. Produces phosphorus crystals on the film.

24. **B**

25. How do you change from a low-contrast film to a high-contrast film and still maintain density?

    A. Decrease the kVp and increase the mAs.
    B. Decrease the kVp and the mAs.
    C. Increase the kVp and decrease the mAs.
    D. Increase the kVp and the mAs.

25. **A**

26. With reference to low kVp units versus high kVp units, which of the following statements is true?

    A. 50 kVp produces short-scale, high-contrast film with many shades of gray.
    B. 50 kVp produces long-scale, high-contrast film with few shades of gray.
    C. 90 kVp produces long-scale, low-contrast film with many shades of gray.
    D. 90 kVp produces long-scale, high-contrast film with few shades of gray.

26. **C**

27. What new mA would be required to reduce the exposure time from 1 second to 0.5 second and maintain the same film density if the original mA were 10?

27. **D**

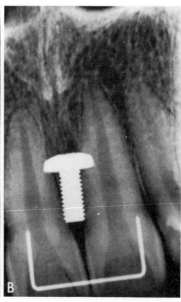

FIGURE 7–9. Two projection techniques. *A,* short-cone. *B,* long-cone.

A. 5 mA.
B. 10 mA.
C. 15 mA.
D. 20 mA.
E. None of the above.

28. The two films in Figure 7–9 were taken in the same manner except a short cone was used for Film A and a long cone was used for Film B. Using the inverse square law, the exposure time (mAs factor) was increased to compensate for the longer cone length. Measure the width of the staple and the length of the screw in Films A and B.

A. With which projection technique has the magnification increased the most? (A) _____.
B. Compare the small screw and staple images. With which technique has better definition been achieved? (B) _____.
C. In which radiograph is the penumbra larger? (C) _____.

28.
A. **Short-cone (Film A)**
B. **Long-cone (Film B)**
C. **Short cone (Film A)**

29. The three films in Figure 7–10 were taken using the paralleling (P), modified paralleling (MP), and bisecting-angle (BA) techniques respectively. The tooth is made of wax impregnated with a barium radiopaque material. A file was inserted to the apex of each root and was not moved between radiographs.

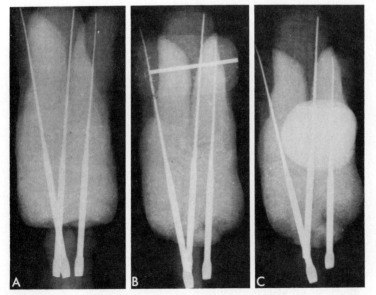

FIGURE 7–10. Three projection techniques. *A*, paralleling (P). *B*, modified paralleling (MP). *C*, bisecting-angle (BA).

A. With which technique is there the most foreshortening? (A) _____.

B. With which technique does the relationship of the files to the apex of the roots appear to change most? (B) _____.

C. With which technique is there the greatest dimensional distortion? (C) _____.

29.
A. Bisecting-angle technique (Film C)
B. Bisecting-angle technique (Film C)
C. Bisecting-angle technique (Film C)

30. The two films in Figure 7–11 were taken using the two most common techniques. Film A was taken using the paralleling technique and a long cone, whereas Film B

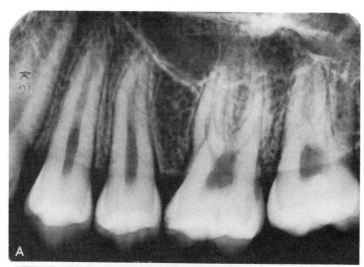

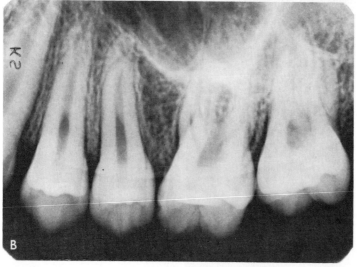

FIGURE 7–11. The two most common projection techniques. *A*, paralleling technique with a long cone. *B*, bisecting-angle technique with a short cone.

was taken using the bisecting-angle technique and a short cone. Compare the two radiographs using the following check list.

	Long-Cone (Paralleling)		Short-Cone (Bisecting-angle)	
	(Yes)	(No)	(Yes)	(No)
Superimposition of buccal and lingual cusps				
Superimposition of buccal portion of alveolar crest with lingual portion of alveolar crest				
Superimposition of zygoma over apices of molar roots				
Contacts of teeth are open				
Maximum image sharpness (definition) of all structures				
Minimal magnification of teeth				
Minimal foreshortening of buccal roots of molars				
Adequate periapical coverage				

Which radiograph reveals the greatest anatomic accuracy? _____.

30. Long cone (paralleling) (Film A)

SECTION 8

LOCALIZATION TECHNIQUES

Olaf E. Langland

CLARK'S RULE

This rule was first described by C. Clark in 1909. It is used to determine the location of foreign objects and impacted or unerupted teeth within the jaws.

The rule requires two periapical radiographs of the area in question. The vertical angulation is fixed for each exposure, whereas the horizontal angulation is varied (see Figure 8–1).

If the foreign object or unerupted tooth <u>moves in the same direction</u> as the horizontal shift of the tube, <u>the object is lingual to the remaining teeth within the jaws.</u> If the object moves in the opposite direction of the tube, the object is buccal or labial to the remaining teeth within the jaws.

BUCCAL-OBJECT RULE

This method of localization was suggested by Richards in 1952 as a way of localizing the mandibular canal. The buccal-object rule can be stated as follows: a buccal object will move with the angulation change of the cone (up or down, left or right). With this technique, the relationship of the apices of the mandibular third molar and the mandibular canal can be estimated (see Figure 8–2). Two radiographs are needed: (1) a

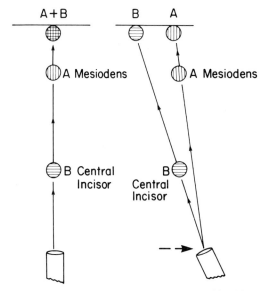

Tube Shift Localization Technique
(Clark's Rule)

FIGURE 8–1. In the tube shift localization technique (Clark's rule), the most lingual object (mesiodens in this case) will move in the same direction as the shift of the tube relative to the more buccal object.

Buccal-Object Rule

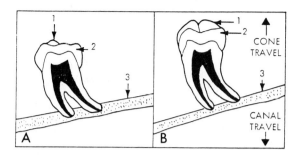

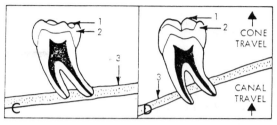

FIGURE 8-2. *A,* Taken with 0° vertical angulation. *B,* Taken with −20° vertical angulation. Canal moves opposite to cone travel and is lingual to tooth. *C,* Taken with 0° vertical angulation. *D,* Taken with −20° vertical angulation. Canal moves with cone travel and is buccal to tooth. 1 = buccal cusp tip; 2 = lingual cusp tip; 3 = mandibular canal. (From O. E., Langland and F. M. Sippy, Textbook of Dental Radiography, Revised 1st Edition, 1975, Courtesy of Charles C Thomas, Publisher, Springfield, Illinois.)

routine view of the mandibular third molar using 0° vertical angulation, and (2) a view with a −20° change in vertical angulation.

If the mandibular canal moves in a direction superior to the apices of the third molar, the mandibular canal is buccal to the third molar. If the mandibular canal moves in a direction inferior to the apices of the third molar, the mandibular canal is lingual to the third molar. If the mandibular canal does not appear to move, it is in the same plane as the third molar.

Sample Examination Questions

1. The three radiographs in Figure 8–3 are part of a full mouth series taken on a dried specimen (skull). On the basis of Clark's rule, the mesiodens is located _____ _____.

    1. lingually (The tube is shifted from the patient's right to the left and the mesiodens moves in the same direction.)

2. The application of Clark's rule obviates the necessity of a (A) _____ view, which exposes the patient to a higher (B)_____.

    2.
    A. maxillary crossfire
    B. radiation dose

3. In this dried specimen (Figure 8–4), one triangle and one diamond shape were placed on either the buccal or lingual cortical plate. A stainless steel wire was also placed in the mandibular canal.

    Film A was taken with a vertical angulation of 0°, and Film B was taken with a vertical angulation of −20°. Using the buccal-object rule, the triangle is (A) _____ _____ to the apices of the third molar, whereas the diamond shape is (B) _____ _____. The mandibular canal is just slightly (C)_____ _____ to the roots of the mandibular third molar.

    3.
    A. buccal (Note that for a −20° angulation the triangle moved upward.)
    B. lingual (The diamond shape moved in the opposite direction of the tip of the cone.)

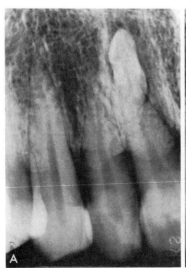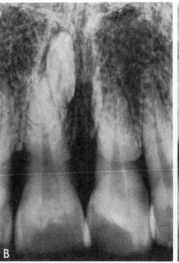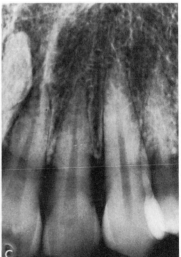

FIGURE 8–3

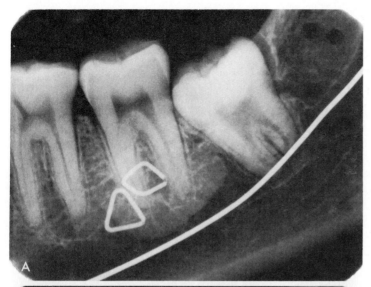

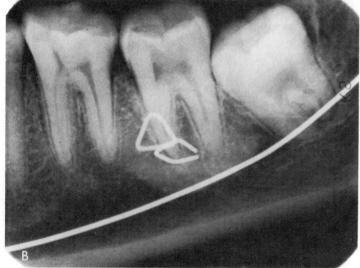

FIGURE 8-4

C. buccal (The wire
moved up slightly from
Film A to Film B. There-
fore, it moved with the
direction of the tip of the
cone.)

4. Which of the following projections would be required to
aid localization of an impacted maxillary bicuspid after
disclosure by an adequate periapical examination?

4. D

A. Waters projection.
B. Cephalometric projection.
C. PA projection of the skull.
D. Maxillary occlusal projection.

5. The localization rule whereby the lingual object follows the movement of the radiation source (tube head) is known as:

   A. Clark's rule.
   B. Rapier's technique.
   C. Miller's technique.
   D. Richards' technique.

6. The localization rule whereby the buccal object follows the movement of the tip of the cone is known as the buccal-object rule and was first described in 1952 by _____.

   A. Rapier.
   B. Miller.
   C. Richards.
   D. Clark.

7. The localization technique, used mainly in the anterior area, whereby an ordinary periapical film is taken followed by an extraoral lateral view at right angles to the object is called the _____ technique.
   (1) Langland.
   (2) Sippy.
   (3) Miller.
   (4) Right-angle.

   A. 2.
   B. 3.
   C. 1 and 2.
   D. 3 and 4.

8. The *SLOB* rule usually refers to _____ rule and stands for *S*ame on *L*ingual; *O*pposite on *B*uccal.

   A. Miller's.
   B. Clark's.
   C. Richards'.
   D. Kasle's.

9. Which of the following most accurately describes the amount of image shift of buccally oriented objects (as compared to lingually oriented objects) when the horizontal or vertical angle of the x-ray beam changes?

   A. Minimum shift.
   B. Maximum shift.
   C. Depends on whether the film and the object are parallel or if they form an angle.
   D. Depends on whether the vertical or horizontal angle is changed.
   E. Equal amount of shifting for each.

5. A

6. C

7. D

8. B

9. B

SECTION 9

INTRAORAL
EXPOSURE TECHNIQUES

This volume would not be complete if we did not review the principles of the two most commonly used intraoral exposure techniques. They are the (1) _____ and the (2) _____ techniques.

Look at Figure 9–1 and you will see that in the bisecting-angle technique the principle is to place the film as close to the tooth as possible; the central ray of the x-ray beam is then directed perpendicular to (3) _____ _____.

In the paralleling technique (Figure 9–2), the film is placed parallel to the long axis of the tooth, and the central ray is directed perpendicular to (4) _____.

In the bisecting-angle technique, digital retention of the film by the patient is usually used for (5) _____ teeth, whereas bite blocks are usually used for the (6) _____ teeth. In the paralleling technique, some sort of bite block with an attached external (7) _____ _____ device is preferred.

Two intraoral exposures whereby there are minimal differences in the images produced by the two exposure techniques are in the (8) _____ and (9) _____ areas.

This is because the (10) _____ of most patients is such that the film will be placed (11) _____ to the long axis of the teeth regardless of which technique is used.

Generally, pointed cones are undesirable because of (12) _____. In fact, the use of pointed cones is now prohibited in (13) _____. Open-ended cones are more desirable than (14) _____ cones. What about long cones versus short cones? From study-

1. bisecting-angle
2. paralleling

3. an imaginary plane halfway between the angle formed by the long axis of the tooth and the plane of the film
4. the plane of the film
5. upper

6. lower
7. cone-positioning or collimating

8. mandibular bicuspid
9. mandibular molar

10. anatomy
11. parallel

12. scatter radiation caused by the interaction of the x rays with the material at the tip of the cone
13. the manufacture of new equipment
14. pointed

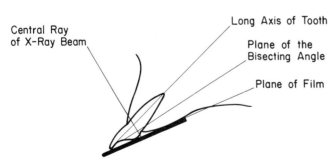

Central Ray of X-Ray Beam

Long Axis of Tooth

Plane of the Bisecting Angle

Plane of Film

Bisecting–Angle Technique

FIGURE 9–1.

ing the inverse square law you know that if the milliamperage and kVp remain constant, the exposure time will quadruple if the length of the cone is doubled. Therefore, the patient will receive (15) _____ radiation exposure at
the skin. Because the diameter of the beam emerging from
the long cone is (16) _____ than that of the short
cone, a (17) _____ volume of the patient's tissues is
irradiated. The (18) _____ cone exposes the
patient to the least amount of radiation.

Whether you are using the bisecting-angle or the paralleling
technique, the preferred cone length is (19) _____ inches.
Can you name three advantages of the long cone over the
short cone? (20–22) _____, _____
_____, and _____.
Can you name four advantages of the paralleling technique
using the position-indicating device over the bisecting-angle
technique? (23–26) _____, _____
_____, _____. and
_____.

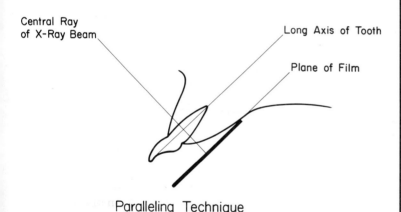

Central Ray
of X-Ray Beam

Long Axis of Tooth

Plane of Film

Paralleling Technique

FIGURE 9–2.

When does the long round cone expose the same amount of
tissue as the long rectangular cone? (27)_____
_____.

15. the same

16. smaller
17. smaller
18. rectangular

19. 16
20. less object magni-
    fication
21. reduction of pen-
    umbra, thereby in-
    creasing object
    sharpness and
    detail
22. smaller beam of
    radiation, thereby
    reducing the dose
    to the patient
23. minimal elongation
    and foreshortening
    of the object
24. less dimensional
    distortion (elonga-
    tion of the palatal
    roots and foreshort-
    ening of the buccal
    roots of maxillary
    molars)
25. anatomic accuracy
    (For example, the
    malar process is not
    superimposed on
    the apices of the
    maxillary molars.)
26. positive alignment
    of the beam, film,
    and object
27. When the extraoral
    beam-positioning
    and collimating de-
    vice is used.

Sample Examination Questions

1. The long-cone or paralleling technique is advised because we can:

    A. Use the shorter time intervals allowable with an electronic timer.
    B. Use a longer focal spot–film distance to compensate for a greater object-film distance, to reduce magnification and distortion.
    C. Hold the film closer to the tooth so there is less magnification and a better image.
    D. Use a lower kVp.
    E. B and C.

    1. B

2. The advantage of the paralleling technique over the bisecting-angle technique is:

    A. The increased anatomic accuracy of the radiographic image.
    B. The increased object-film distance.
    C. The greater magnification of the image.
    D. That the central ray is perpendicular to an imaginary line drawn through half the angle between the long axis of the teeth and the film.

    2. A

3. The paralleling technique is recommended over the bisecting-angle technique because:

    A. Positioning the film is easier.
    B. It uses slower film.
    C. It gives a less distorted picture of the length of the root.
    D. It cuts developing time.
    E. A, B, and C.

    3. C

4. Why is the extension or long cone a necessary adjunct to the paralleling technique?

    A. To avoid magnification of the image.
    B. To avoid shape distortion of the image.
    C. To reduce secondary radiation.
    D. To facilitate correct vertical angulation of the cone.
    E. To avoid superimposition of structures.

    4. A

5. What is the main cause of foreshortening in the bisecting-angle technique?

   A. Improper placement of the film.
   B. Improper horizontal angulation of the cone.
   C. Vertical angulation of the cone is too obtuse.
   D. Vertical angulation of the cone is too acute or sharp.

6. Compared with the short-cone (bisecting-angle) technique, the right-angle (paralleling) technique using the extension cones involves:

   (1) Greater vertical angulations.
   (2) Greater object-film distances.
   (3) Shorter developing times.
   (4) Greater anode-film distances.
   A. 1 and 2.
   B. 1 and 3.
   C. 2 and 3.
   D. 2 and 4.
   E. 3 and 4.

7. Your x-ray machine has a short pointed cone. Which radiographic technique would be most appropriate to use?

   A. Paralleling.
   B. Right-angle.
   C. Bisecting-angle.
   D. Modified.

8. Which statement is most correct?

   A. The long cone can be used with either the paralleling or the bisecting-angle technique.
   B. The long cone is used with the paralleling technique only.
   C. The short cone is used with either the paralleling or the bisecting-angle technique.
   D. Film holders are not necessary with the paralleling technique.

9. With the paralleling technique, it is important to use:

   A. A short target-film distance to avoid loss of detail.
   B. A short cone to decrease magnification.
   C. A long target-film distance to increase magnification.
   D. A long target-film distance to decrease the penumbra.

5. D

6. D

7. C

8. A

9. D

10. In the paralleling technique, the most accurate image of a tooth is produced on the radiograph when the central ray is:

   A. 30° to the long axis of the tooth.
   B. 90° to the film and tooth.
   C. 80° to the plane of the x ray.
   D. 90° to a plane bisecting the long axis of the tooth and the plane of the x ray.

11. The technique that shows the upper and lower crowns on the same radiograph is called the:

   A. Bisecting-angle technique.
   B. Bite-wing technique.
   C. Paralleling technique.
   D. Occlusal technique.

12. When bite-wing x rays are taken without an alignment instrument, the midsagittal plane of the patient's head should be:

   A. Parallel to the floor.
   B. Parallel to the tube.
   C. Perpendicular to the floor.
   D. Perpendicular to the tube.

13. X-ray intensity (I), like light, is related to its distance (D) from the source. This is expressed as the inverse square law and is formulated as:

$$\frac{I_1}{I_2} = \frac{(D_2)^2}{(D_1)^2}$$

If the distance from the source to the object is tripled, the intensity of the x-ray beam at the new distance (D_2) would be:

   A. One-ninth the original distance (D_1).
   B. One-sixth the original distance.
   C. One-third the original distance.
   D. One-half the original distance.

14. The intensity of x-radiation at any given distance from the source of radiation varies:

    A. Inversely with the square of the distance.
    B. Directly with the square of the distance.
    C. Inversely with the distance.
    D. Directly with the distance.

14. A

15. When an 8-inch target-film distance is changed to a 16-inch target-film distance (kV and mA kept constant), the exposure time should be:

    A. Doubled.
    B. Decreased by half.
    C. Increased by half.
    D. Quadrupled.

15. D

$$\frac{I_1}{I_2} = \frac{(D_2)^2}{(D_1)^2} \quad \frac{16 \times 16}{8 \times 8} = 4$$

16. A dentist uses the following factors in making a radiograph of the maxillary incisor region: FFD = 8 inches; kVp = 65; mA = 10; time = .75 second. He wishes to change to a long-cone technique (FFD = 16 inches) employing 15 mA. What would his new exposure time be?

    A. 1 second.
    B. 2 seconds.
    C. 3 seconds.
    D. 4 seconds.
    E. None of the above.

16. B

17. If a satisfactory radiograph was produced using a target-film distance of 8 inches and an exposure time of 1 second, what would be the correct exposure time for a target-film distance of 16 inches?

    A. 2 seconds.
    B. 4 seconds.
    C. 6 seconds.
    D. 8 seconds.

17. B

18. At 90 kVp and 15 mA at a cone distance of 8 inches, the exposure time for a film is .50 second. In the same situation, the exposure time at 16 inches would be:

    A. 0.25 second.
    B. 1.00 second.
    C. 2.00 seconds.
    D. 4.00 seconds.

18. C

19. The radiation output of a machine at a 16-inch source-film distance is 250 mR per second. Under identical exposure conditions, if the source-film distance is changed to 12 inches, what will be the new output per second?

    A. 140 mR.
    B. 200 mR.
    C. 333 mR.
    D. 444 mR.

[handwritten: 16inch 250mR / 12inch <250]

[handwritten: $\frac{I_1}{I_2} = \frac{16 \times 16}{12 \times 12} = \frac{16}{3}$, $\frac{3}{16} \times 250 = \frac{750}{16}$, $16\overline{)750}$]

20. A dentist is currently using 90 kVp, 15 mA, 2.50 mm Al filtration, and 0.20-second exposure time. His radiation source-film distance is 8 inches. He decides to change the radiation source–film distance to 12 inches. What should be the new exposure time?

    A. 0.09 second.
    B. 0.30 second.
    C. 0.45 second.
    D. 11.20 seconds.

[handwritten: $\frac{I_1}{I_2} = \frac{12 \times 12}{8 \times 8} = \frac{9}{4}$]

21. If the distance for an exposure was 2 feet and the exposure time was 1 second, what would be the exposure time if the distance was changed to 6 feet if the film density is to remain constant?

    A. 3 seconds.
    B. 4 seconds.
    C. 6 seconds.
    D. 9 seconds.

22. If the focal spot–object distance is 8 inches, kVp is 65, mA is 10, exposure time is 12 impulses, and the resulting radiograph is acceptable, what should be the exposure time if the distance is changed to 16 inches?

    A. 3 impulses.
    B. 6 impulses.
    C. 24 impulses.
    D. 48 impulses.

23. As used in intraoral radiography, the bisecting-angle technique is one in which the central x-ray beam is directed:

    A. Perpendicular to the long axis of the object.
    B. Parallel to the long axis of the object.
    C. Perpendicular to a line bisecting the angle formed by the object and the film packet.
    D. Perpendicular to the long plane of the film packet.

SECTION 10

FILM, CASSETTES, AND INTENSIFYING SCREENS

INTRAORAL FILM, CASSETTES, AND INTENSIFYING SCREENS

Look at Figure 10–1 and name the layers that make up the
Film: (1–A) _____ , (B) _____ ,
(C) _____ , (D) _____ .
Note that the intraoral film consists of a (2) _____
emulsion, which in turn consists of a thin layer of (3)
_____ containing (4) _____ crystals. These crystals are often referred to as the (5)____
_____ of the film, and the size of these crystals determines
the (6) _____ of the film. The larger the size of the
(7) _____ , the (8) _____ the film speed.
The (9) _____ base is a (10) _____ tint,
and the protective outer coating is (11) _____ .

Look at Figure 10–2 and identify the components that make
up the intraoral film packet: (12–A) _____
_____ , (B) _____ , (C) _____
_____ , (D) _____ , (E)
_____ , (F) _____ , (G) _____
_____ . Note that the (13) _____ is located on
the (14) _____ side of the packet. When the film is
placed in the mouth, the (15) _____ side of the

1.
A. acetate base
B. adhesive layer or
    substratum
C. emulsion
D. protective layer
2. double
3. gelatin
4. silver bromide
5. grain
6. speed
7. grain
8. faster
9. acetate
10. bluish
11. clear
12.
A. dot locator (on tab
    side of packet)
B. convex surface of
    the dot
C. outer wrapping (soft
    plastic or paper)
D. inner film wrapping
E. film
F. lead backing
G. printed, colored, or
    tab side of the packet
13. dot
14. tab (printed,
    colored, back)
15. plain

Intraoral Film

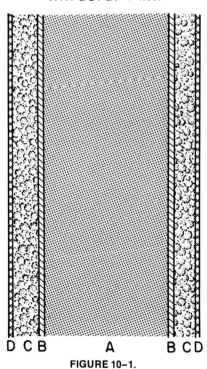

D C B   A   B C D

FIGURE 10–1.

Intraoral Film Packet

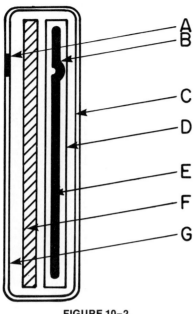

FIGURE 10–2.

packet should face toward the teeth and the source of radiation, with the dot oriented toward the (16) _____ surfaces of the teeth. One exception to this rule is the (17) _____ view. Therefore, when trying to orient the the right and left sides of the patient upon mounting the films, it is important to remember that the (18) _____ surface of the dot faces the source of radiation. This also means that as you look at the film with the convex surface of the dot oriented towards you, the patient's right side will be on your (19) _____ side and vice versa for the patient's left side.

Now look at Figure 10–3 and think of the convex surface or "bulge" side of the dot as pointing the same way as the patient's nose. Therefore, if you are looking at the bulge side of the dot, the patient's right side will be on your (20) _____ side; if, however, you are looking at the concave side of the dot, as you would if you were sitting on the patient's tongue, the patient's right side would be on your (21) _____.
It is therefore important to orient the dot properly when mounting the film so that the right and left sides do not get mixed up. If the back of the film packet faces the source of radiation, a (22) _____ pattern will show up on the processed film. Such films should never be used because (1) they will be of poor diagnostic quality and (2) the orientation of the dot will be such that the patient's right and left sides will be (23) _____.

16. **occlusal (incisal)**
17. **bite-wing**

18. **convex**

19. **left**

20. **left**

21. **right**

22. **herringbone or tire track**

23. **reversed**

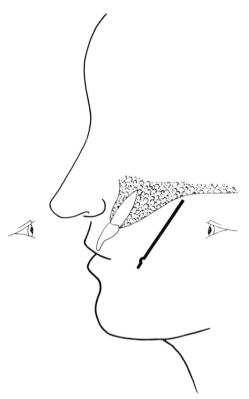

FIGURE 10–3. Positioning of intraoral film packet.

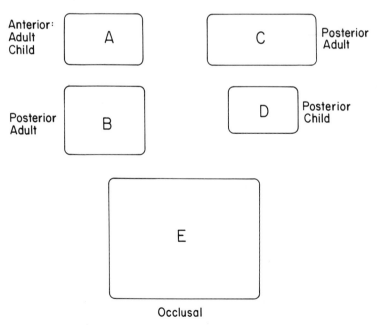

FIGURE 10–4. Relative size of intraoral films.

Anterior: Adult Child — A

Posterior Adult — C

Posterior Adult — B

Posterior Child — D

Occlusal — E

Each of the intraoral films identified in Figure 10–4 has a numerical size. Identify the size of each: (24–A) _____, (B) _____, (C) _____, (D) _____, (E) _____.

In addition to the previously mentioned intraoral nonscreen films, a 5 × 7 inch extraoral nonscreen film is also available and is most commonly used for the (25) _____ and (26) _____ views.

25. lateral jaw (body of the mandible)
26. lateral ramus

EXTRAORAL FILM, CASSETTES, AND INTENSIFYING SCREENS

A significant difference between intraoral and extraoral films is that the former is more sensitive to (27) _____, whereas the latter is more sensitive to (28)_____ _____. Extraoral films, therefore, require a vehicle or medium whereby the radiant energy of incoming x rays can be converted into (29) _____.

27. x rays
28. fluorescent light

29. fluorescent light

This is accomplished by sandwiching the extraoral film between two (30) _____ that contain (31) _____, which fluoresce in the presence of (32) _____. This type of film is most commonly referred to as (33) _____ film. Refer to Figure 10–5 and be certain that you know the layers of the screens and film.

30. intensifying screens
31. calcium tungstate or other suitable phosphors
32. x-radiation
33. screen

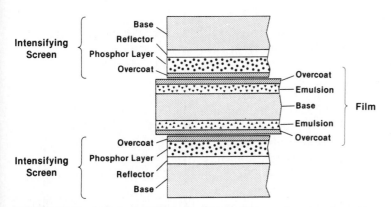

FIGURE 10–5. Screen and film layers. (From "Screen Imaging, Image Insight 3 Workbook." Published by Health Sciences Markets Division, Eastman Kodak Company, Rochester, NY.)

The packet containing the screen film is called a (34) _____ _____. It consists of a front surface easily penetrable by (35) _____. Beneath this is the intensifying screen containing the fluorescent phosphors. Next is the film, and immediately beneath this is another intensifying screen. The film is pressed into firm contact between and with the two screens by the back cover, which is closed under pressure. The speed of such cassettes depends on the thickness of the (36) __ _____ in the screen. The greater the (37) _____, the greater the loss of definition and the lesser the amount of (38) _____ _____ required. Therefore, fast screens require less (39) _____, but there is some loss of (40) _____ in the image. Conversely, slow screens require more (41) _____, and a higher (42) _____ image is produced. Generally, screen films require (43) _____ x-radiation than nonscreen films for diagnostic-quality radiographs. One of the disadvantages of extraoral cassettes in skull radiography is the (44) _____ caused by the secondary radiation produced. This can be overcome by using (45) _____. In dentistry, the (46) _____ is generally incorporated into the front of the (47) _____. This produces a number of horizontal opaque lines on the radiographic image. When the use of a grid is considered desirable but the horizontal grid lines on the image are considered undesirable, a (48) _____ grid may be used. Generally, grids require (49) _____ radiation.

Thus far you may have been led to believe that, apart from the density of the structures being radiographed, the amount of radiation required to adequately expose a screen film depends on the (50) _____ and whether or not (51) _____ are used. Assuming that the film speed and other factors are kept constant, the idea is to increase the speed of the screen with a minimal loss of (52) _____ in the image using a (53) _____ amount of x-radiation. Can you name five other factors that influence the speed of the screen and the effect of each on the sharpness of the image? (See Figure 10–6.) Recently, the introduction of rare-earth screens has produced a (54) _____ reduction in the amount of radiation needed to produce diagnostic-quality radiographs as compared with traditional screens. These screens contain phosphors of the lanthanide series of elements such as (55) _____ _____. These rare-earth phosphors produce a (56) _____ fluorescence and, therefore, a compatible (57) _____-sensitive x-ray screen film must be used. Additionally, the use of such film requires the replacement of the (58) _____ in the darkroom.

34. cassette
35. x rays
36. phosphor layer
37. thickness of the phosphor layer
38. x-radiation
39. x-radiation
40. definition
41. x-radiation
42. definition
43. much less
44. fog
45. grids
46. grid
47. cassette
48. reciprocating or moving
49. more
50. thickness of the phosphor layer
51. grids
52. sharpness and detail
53. minimal
54. significant
55. gadolinium oxysulfide
56. green
57. green
58. safelight filter (e.g., Kodak GBX filter)

Remember also that cassettes containing intensifying screens are used in panoramic radiography. These may be flat or curved or rigid or nonrigid, and (59) _____ screens may be used.

59. rare-earth

Factor	Major influence on:	
	Speed	Sharpness
X-ray absorption of phosphor	Increases—uses more of available x-rays.	No influence. Does not increase quantum mottle.
Light output per absorption event	Increases—more light available to film.	No direct influence. Increase in quantum mottle.
Absorption of light in phosphor layer	Decreases—allows less light to impinge on film.	Increases—reduces light spread of disc image.
Thickness of phosphor layer	Increases—uses more of available x-rays.	Decreases—poorer screen geometry.
Reflecting layer	Increases—makes more use of light from crystal available to film.	Decreases—poorer screen geometry.
Size of crystal	Increases.	Decreases.
Asymmetry of screen	Minor effect.	Increases—brings areas of greater absorption closer to film. Improved geometry.
Reduction of cross-over—shift of screen emission to UV	Minor effect.	Increases due to better geometry.

FIGURE 10–6. Factors influencing the speed of the screen. The effects of the imaging properties of the film-screen combination on quantum mottle are not included. (From "Screen Imaging, Image Insight 3 Workbook." Published by Health Sciences Markets Division, Eastman Kodak Company, Rochester, NY.)

Sample Examination Questions

1. Which of the following is the correct description of intensifying screens?

    A. Thinner phosphor layers result in faster screens.
    B. Thinner phosphor layers result in more unsharpness.
    C. Thicker phosphor layers result in faster screens.
    D. Thicker phosphor layers result in less unsharpness.

    1. C

2. Which of the following best describes a slow-speed intensifying screen as compared with a fast-speed intensifying screen?

    A. Thick phosphor layers produce an unsharp image.
    B. Thick phosphor layers produce a sharp image.
    C. Thin phosphor layers produce an unsharp image.
    D. Thin phosphor layers produce a sharp image.

    2. D

3. Cone-cutting (partial image) on a radiograph is caused by:

    A. Underexposure.
    B. Improper exposure technique.
    C. A damaged cone.
    D. Improper coverage of the film with the beam of radiation.

    3. D

4. A cassette:

    A. Emits light.
    B. Is a container for film and screens.
    C. Is an instrument to align the x-ray cone.
    D. Records the patient's exposure.

    4. B

5. A herringbone pattern appears on a film if it is:

    A. Not processed properly.
    B. Given too much radiation.
    C. Not exposed to a sufficient amount of radiation.
    D. Placed in the oral cavity backwards.

    5. D

6. Grids result in:

    (1)   Less radiation to the patient.
    (2)   More radiation to the patient.
    (3)   Less contrast.
    (4)   More contrast.
  A. 1 and 4.
  B. 1 and 3.
  C. 2 and 3.
  D. 2 and 4.

6. D

7. A grid is:

  A. Used to focus a beam of electrons on the focal spot.
  B. Used to limit the size of the beam and reduce radiation exposure.
  C. Never used because it has insignificant effects.
  D. Used to reduce scatter radiation to the film.
  E. Used to reduce the patient exposure to x rays by removing deflected photons.

7. D

8. A latent image is:

  A. An image that is very late in its formation.
  B. A very light radiographic image.
  C. Produced after exposure but before developing.
  D. A very dark radiographic image.

8. C

9. The primary reason for using fast films is to:

  A. Save time in the dental office.
  B. Give a better image quality.
  C. Reduce the radiation dose to the patient.
  D. Reduce the processing time.

9. C

10. Intensifying screens are used with extraoral films to:

  A. Increase the exposure time.
  B. Improve image quality.
  C. Decrease radiation to the patient.
  D. Increase the kVp.

10. C

11. When a standard dental x-ray film is exposed to a diagnostic dose of radiation, only a small portion of the radiation is absorbed by the film emulsion. The amount of radiation absorbed by the film is approximately:

    A. 2%.
    B. 4%.
    C. 8%.
    D. 12%.

12. The use of high-speed radiographic film:

    (1) Can reduce radiation to the patient.
    (2) Cannot reduce radiation to the patient.
    (3) Increases radiation scatter.
    (4) Increases image sharpness.
    A. 1.
    B. 3.
    C. 4.
    D. 1 and 4.
    E. 2 and 4.

13. The characteristic (Hurter & Driffield) curve of an x-ray film:

    (1) Depends on the amount of light transmitted through it.
    (2) Depends on the thickness of the film emulsion.
    (3) Is different for each film and is a quality of the emulsion.
    (4) Depends on the time the measuring light is passed through the film.
    A. 1 and 2.
    B. 2 and 3.
    C. 3 and 4.
    D. 1 and 4.
    E. None of the above.

14. Which of the following is *NOT* a reason for using Speed D dental film?

    A. To reduce motion unsharpness.
    B. To increase image quality.
    C. To decrease exposure time.
    D. To reduce radiation to the patient.

15. The efficiency with which a film responds to x-ray exposure is known as film sensitivity or, more commonly, speed. Which speed range is best for reducing radiation to the patient?

    A. Speed A.
    B. Speed B.
    C. Speed C.
    D. Speed D.

15. D

16. Nonscreen extraoral films have to be developed in manual tanks (not in automatic processors) because they:

    A. Are more sensitive to x rays than to light.
    B. Have large silver bromide crystals.
    C. Have a thicker emulsion than screen films.
    D. Do not require screens for exposing a film.

16. C

17. What is the function of the raised dot on the dental film?

    A. It identifies the side of film toward the line of occlusion.
    B. It identifies the side of the film toward the tongue.
    C. It identifies the side of the film toward the beam of radiation.
    D. It identifies the maxillary or mandibular teeth, depending on how the film is placed in the mouth.

17. C

18. If a film is stripped from its packet and exposed to light, after processing it will:

    A. Be unaffected.
    B. Turn white.
    C. Turn black.
    D. Be translucent.

18. C

19. Which of the following films can be used intraorally and extraorally?

    A. Screen film.
    B. Occlusal film.
    C. Periapical film.
    D. Bite-wing film.

19. B

20. Which of the following will *NOT* produce film fog? **20. D**

    A. Films left unprotected in the operatory where patients are x-rayed.
    B. Films stored for many years or in an unsafe place.
    C. Light leaks in the darkroom.
    D. Films stored in lead containers.

21. Which of the following will produce film fog? **21. D**

    A. Light leaks in the darkroom.
    B. Films stored for many years or in an unsafe place.
    C. Films left unprotected in the operatory where patients are x-rayed.
    D. All of the above.

22. The purpose of the lead foil in back of the film packet is to: **22. B**

    A. Eliminate film motion.
    B. Absorb the x-rays after image registration on the film.
    C. Prevent film contamination.
    D. All of the above.

23. Screen films are used with intensifying screens because these films are: **23. B**

    A. More sensitive to x rays than to light.
    B. More sensitive to light than to x rays.
    C. Coated with silver sulfide crystals.
    D. Coated with calcium tungstate crystals.

24. Periapical radiographic film packets contain which of the following materials? **24. A**

    (1) Lead foil.
    (2) Cardboard backing.
    (3) Film.
    (4) Intensifying screens.
    (5) Copper foil.
    A. 1 and 3.
    B. 1, 2, and 3.
    C. 1, 3, and 4.
    D. 2, 3, and 4.
    E. 3, 4, and 5.

25. The base material used in dental films is:

    A. Sodium thiosulfate.
    B. Metol.
    C. Cellulose acetate.
    D. Gelatin.

25. C

26. Radiographic film emulsion is:

    A. Cellulose acetate.
    B. Sodium thiosulfate.
    C. Hydroquinone.
    D. Gelatin and silver bromide.
    E. Calcium tungstate.

26. D

27. Most extraoral radiographs are taken with the aid of:

    A. A bite-block film holder.
    B. An intensifying screen.
    C. A pointed x-ray cone.
    D. A cellulose nitrate screen.

27. B

28. Intensifying screens:

    (1) Aid in reducing radiation exposure times.
    (2) Contain calcium tungstate crystals.
    (3) Contain silver bromide crystals.
    (4) Consist of x-ray–penetrable base material.
    A. 2 and 3.
    B. 3 and 4.
    C. 1, 2, and 3.
    D. 1, 2, and 4.
    E. All of the above.

28. D

29. Extraoral films are:

    (1) Used when large areas of the skull need to be radiographed.
    (2) Sometimes loaded in cassettes.
    (3) Often used when fractures of the skull are suspected.
    (4) Used only in conjunction with intensifying screens.
    A. 2 and 4.
    B. 3 and 4.
    C. 1, 2, and 3.
    D. 2, 3, and 4.
    E. All of the above.

29. C

30. Intraoral radiographic films are:

    (1) Occlusal radiographs.
    (2) Cassette-type radiographs.
    (3) Bite-wing radiographs.
    (4) Ready-pack lateral jaw radiographs.
    (5) Periapical radiographs.

A. 1, 2, and 5.
B. 1, 3, and 5.
C. 2, 4, and 5.
D. 3, 4, and 5.
E. 1, 2, 4, and 5.

30. B

31. Unexposed radiographic films:

    (1) Should be stored in a cool, dry place.
    (2) Have an indefinite shelf life.
    (3) Must be protected from heat.
    (4) Deteriorate with age.
    (5) Must be protected from moisture.

A. 1, 2, and 3.
B. 2, 3, and 5.
C. 3, 4, and 5.
D. 1, 2, 3, and 5.
E. 1, 3, 4, and 5.

31. E

32. The film speed is directly related to the:

A. Size of the silver bromide crystals.
B. Amount of radiation required to produce radiographic density.
C. Exposure latitude.
D. None of the above.

32. A

33. A cassette was opened in the darkroom to remove and process the exposed film. A piece of black paper was discovered on the surface of the intensifying screen. The paper most likely would produce:

A. A white or light artifact.
B. A black artifact.
C. No artifact.
D. Reticulation.

33. A

34. Gelatin is a good radiographic emulsion vehicle because it:

    A. Enhances contrast.
    B. Is soluble in water at temperatures required for processing.
    C. Is chemically inert.
    D. Undergoes volumetric changes during film exposures.

34. C

35. Sensitization specks:

    A. Are defects in calcium tungstate crystals.
    B. Are defects in silver bromide crystals.
    C. Act as electron traps.
    D. A and C.
    E. B and C.

35. E

SECTION 11

THE CHEMISTRY OF IMAGE
PRODUCTION AND PROCESSING

TABLE 11-1. PROCESSING SOLUTIONS AND THEIR FUNCTIONS

Developer	Fixer
Developing (reducing) agents (reduce exposed grains of Ag in AgBr to free metallic Ag) 　Elon or Metol – stable, works quickly, brings out grays 　Hydroquinone – unstable, works slowly, brings out blacks and whites **Preservative** (prevents rapid oxidation of unstable developing agents) 　Sodium sulfite – an anti-oxidant **Accelerator** (activates the developing agents, softens the emulsion) 　Sodium carbonate – an alkali **Restrainer** (restrains the developing agents from developing or reducing unexposed grains of Ag, thus producing fog) 　Potassium bromide **Solvent** (vehicle for developer chemicals; softens gelatin emulsion) 　Water	**Fixing (clearing) agent** (removes undeveloped AgBr from emulsion; requires several minutes; after clearing, film may be wet-read) 　Sodium thiosulfate – hyposulfite **Preservative** (prevents chemical breakdown of fixing agent) 　Sodium sulfite **Acidifier** (provides acid pH required by the hardener; neutralizes any remaining alkaline developer) 　Acetic acid – an acid **Hardener** (shrinks and hardens the soft, swollen gelatin emulsion) 　Potassium alum – requires acid pH **Solvent** (vehicle for fixer chemicals) 　Water

To understand processing solutions, it is first necessary to become familiar with the components of the solutions and their functions. The best way to do this is to familiarize yourself with Table 11-1.

Now that you have done this, label Figure 11-1 (1) _____ _____, Figure 11-2 (2) _____ _____, and Figure 11-3 (3) _____ _____.

1. exposed film containing the latent image
2. developed but unfixed image
3. fixed image

Remember that the idea of processing the film is to render the latent or invisible image visible. The latent image consists of (4) _____, whereas the processed image is nothing more than (5) _____ _____.

4. exposed silver bromide crystals
5. a bunch of small black specks or grains of silver with the remaining halide and unexposed silver bromide crystals removed

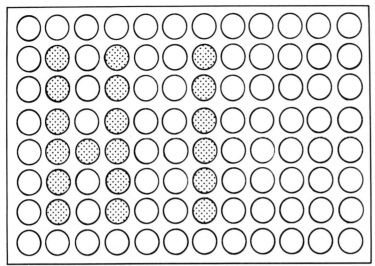

FIGURE 11-1.

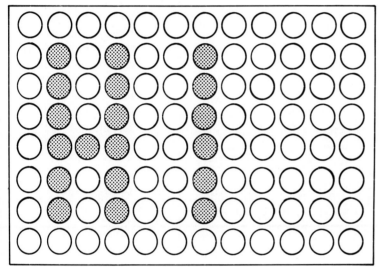

FIGURE 11-2.

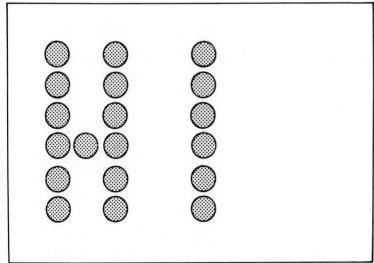

FIGURE 11-3.

To review the whole sequence: the first thing that happens to the silver bromide crystal is that a tiny "latent-image center" consisting of neutral silver atoms is formed as a result of (6) _____. Then the film is brought into the darkroom, where it may be further exposed by (7) _____

_____

or a (8) _____. The developing solution (9) _____ the exposed silver bromide to (10) _____ Next, the film is rinsed in water to (11) _____ and is then placed into the fixer. This step is necessary to (12) _____ any unexposed silver bromide crystals. Finally, the free silver, which is contained within the emulsion and which forms the image, is (13) _____ for approximately (14) _____ minutes. The purpose of this step is to (15) _____

_____ .

6. radiation
7. **An unsafe safelight (e.g., an improper filter, filter too close to the working surface, cracked filter, scratched filter, filter bulb too bright)**
8. **darkroom that is not light-tight**
9. reduces
10. free silver
11. **remove and neutralize the alkaline developer**
12. **clear or remove**
13. washed
14. 20
15. **wash out any remaining chemicals, especially the fixer, which if retained may cause the image to fade or discolor**

It is important to determine how long to place the films in each solution during hand processing. Remember that developing and fixing times depend on the (16) _____ _____ of the solutions used. Therefore, look at Table 11–2 and be sure that you understand this time-temperature relationship. (Remember that the water bath is constantly draining and reaches the desired temperature almost as soon as the water is turned on. Since most developer and fixer tanks contain 1 gallon, they may take up to 1 hour to reach the temperature of the rinse bath. Because developing time determines fixing time, the thermometer should be placed in the developer and checked each time you process.)

16. **temperature**

There are several simple rules to remember with reference to time-temperature developing:

1. Since the temperature of the water bath controls the temperature of the (17) _____ and the (18) _____, the thermometer should be placed in the (19) _____ .

17. **developer**
18. **fixer**
19. **developer**

TABLE 11–2. DEVELOPING AND FIXING TIMES IN MINUTES

Solution Temperature (°F)	Development Time	Rinse	Fixing	Wash
65 (18.5°C)	6	0.5	10–12	20
68 (20°C)	5	0.5	10	20
70 (21°C)	4.5	0.5	9–10	20
72 (22°C)	4	0.5	8–9	20
75 (24°C)	3	0.5	6–7	20
80 (26.5°C)	2.5	0.5	5–6	20

2. Fixing time is approximately (20) _____ times the developing time.

3. Films should not be wet-read until they have (21) _____. This does not usually occur until they have been fixed for at least (22) _____ minutes.

4. Films should not be processed in solutions colder than (23) _____ or warmer than (24) _____, unless otherwise specified by the manufacturer.

5. Films should never be (25) _____ to reduce the developing time or to compensate for worn or depleted (dark yellow or brown) developer.

6. The cardinal rule for successful processing is to read the (26) _____ for all phases of image production.

7. A dirty, messy darkroom usually means (27) _____ films.

There is a simple method of determining whether the developer solution has weakened: when the developing time (28) _____ the recommended time-temperature values. When this occurs, it is important to replenish the developer with developer (29) _____ solution. This solution differs from fresh developer in that it contains greater concentrations of (30) _____ agents; it is more (31) _____ to offset the (32) _____ pH and the restraining action of the (33) _____ that has accumulated.

20.	2
21.	**cleared**
22.	**2**
23.	**65°F (18.5°C)**
24.	**80°F (26.5°C)**
25.	**overexposed**
26.	**manufacturer's instructions**
27.	**poor quality**
28.	**exceeds**
29.	**replenisher**
30.	**developing**
31.	**alkaline**
32.	**decreased**
33.	**bromine**

Sample Examination Questions

1. In the processing of roentgenograms:

    A. Total darkness must be maintained in the dark-room.
    B. The developing solution should be kept as near to room temperature as possible.
    C. You can decrease the time of fixing if the film was overexposed.
    D. Clean, fresh solutions are essential.

    1. **D**

2. Placing the film in the fixer first results in:

    A. A black film.
    B. A clear film.
    C. A mottled film.
    D. No change.

    2. **B**

3. A so-called herringbone pattern results from:

    A. Developer and fixer with different temperatures.
    B. Creasing the film.
    C. Reversing the film to the beam.
    D. Fluoride.

    3. **C**

4. Fluoride contamination of a film from the operator's fingers results in:

    A. White spots.
    B. Black spots.
    C. General increased density.
    D. No change.

    4. **B**

5. Black lines on a film are most likely caused by:

    (1) Creasing.
    (2) High temperature.
    (3) Static electricity.
    (4) Air bubbles.
    A. 1 and 2.
    B. 1 and 3.
    C. 2 and 3.
    D. 3 and 4.

    5. **B**

6. Reticulation occurs when the: 6. C

A. Developer is too hot.
B. Fixer is too cold.
C. Developer and fixer temperatures differ too greatly.
D. Processing procedure takes too long.

7. In the time-temperature processing of dental x-ray films: 7. C

A. Unexposed silver salts are precipitated in the developing solution.
B. The latent image is activated in the fixer bath.
C. Exposed silver salts are precipitated on the film base.
D. The water bath softens the gelatin emulsion.

8. Which of the following reduce the life of the developer solution?   8. D
    (1) Exposure to light.
    (2) Exposure to air.
    (3) Time.
    (4) Heavy use.

A. 1 and 2.
B. 1, 2, and 3.
C. 2, 3, and 4.
D. All of the above.
E. None of the above.

9. Films should be washed in running water for at least: 9. B

A. 10 minutes.
B. 20 minutes.
C. 30 minutes.
D. 40 minutes.

10. The optimum time and temperature for developing film is: 10. D

A. 3 to 4 minutes at 70°F.
B. 4.5 to 5 minutes at 75°F.
C. 4.5 to 5 minutes at 65°F.
D. 4.5 to 5 minutes at 68° to 70°F.

11. Fixing should be:

    (1) Done before developing to produce a harder film.
    (2) Carried out entirely in white light.
    (3) Done at a high temperature.
    (4) Sufficiently long to prevent the image from deteriorating with age (two times developing time).

A. 2.
B. 3.
C. 4.
D. 1 and 4.
E. 2 and 3.

12. Chemical fog on a film is a result of:

    (1) Prolonged exposure of the film to radiation.
    (2) Prolonged development.
    (3) Prolonged washing.
    (4) Prolonged fixing.
    (5) Storage in a cabinet close to other chemicals.

A. 1 and 2.
B. 2 and 3.
C. 2 and 5.
D. 1, 2, 3, and 4.
E. All of the above.

13. To test for chemically or age-fogged film:

A. Develop the film without exposure.
B. Develop the film after exposure.
C. Hold the film up to a bright safelight.
D. Fix the film only.
E. C and D.

14. Slight overdevelopment of a dental film will:

    (1) Not affect its diagnostic acceptability if it has been overexposed.
    (2) Not affect its diagnostic acceptability if it has been properly exposed.
    (3) Affect its diagnostic acceptability if it has been properly exposed.
    (4) Affect its diagnostic acceptability if it has been overexposed.

A. 1.
B. 3.
C. 4.
D. 1 and 3.
E. 2 and 4.

15. The optimum temperature for manual film processing is:

    A. 58°F.
    B. 68°F.
    C. 78°F.
    D. 88°F.

15. **B**

16. The basic developing solution contains:
    (1) Metol.
    (2) Acid.
    (3) Silver bromide.
    (4) Methyl methacrylate.
    (5) Accelerator (alkali).
    (6) Hydrogen peroxide.
    (7) Sodium thiosulfate.
    (8) Aluminum.

    A. 1 and 5.
    B. 1 and 7.
    C. 2 and 7.
    D. 5 and 6.

16. **A**

17. The basic fixing solution contains which of the items listed in Question 16?

    A. 1 and 7.
    B. 1 and 8.
    C. 2 and 7.
    D. 6 and 8.

17. **C**

18. Fixing time for films is usually:

    A. 10 minutes.
    B. 15 minutes.
    C. 20 minutes.
    D. Dependent on temperature.

18. **A**

19. What is the most technical method for developing films?

    A. Visual-temperature method.
    B. Visual method.
    C. Time-temperature method.
    D. Time method.

19. **C**

20. What is the cause of yellow or brown stains appearing on film some months after processing?

   A. Aged film.
   B. Improper exposure technique.
   C. Films stored in a hot place.
   D. Incomplete fixing and washing.

21. Radiographs are rinsed in clean running water to:

   A. Rid the film of chemicals.
   B. Dissolve metallic silver.
   C. Shrink the emulsion.
   D. Get rid of the latent image.

22. Contrast of radiographic images is slowly enhanced by:

   A. Alum.
   B. Hydroquinone.
   C. Sodium acetate.
   D. Sodium sulfate.
   E. Sulfuric acid.

23. Film gelatin is softened in the developer solution by the addition of:

   A. Sodium sulfate.
   B. Hydroquinone.
   C. Acetic acid.
   D. Potassium alum.
   E. Sodium carbonate.

24. Chemical fog is controlled in the developer solution by adding:

   A. Elon.
   B. Acetic acid.
   C. Sodium carbonate.
   D. Potassium bromide.
   E. Sodium sulfite.

25. Unexposed silver crystals dissolve when _____ is added to the fixer solution.

   A. Acetic acid.
   B. Sodium thiosulfate.   *Fixing = Clearing*
   C. Sodium sulfate.
   D. Potassium alum.
   E. Sodium carbonate.

20. D

21. A

22. B

23. E

24. D

25. B

26. Which of the following describes film with silver bromide crystals?

   A. Exposed and fixed.
   B. Unexposed and fixed.
   C. Unexposed, developed, and fixed.
   D. Exposed, developed, and fixed.
   E. None of the above.

26. E

27. A radiographic film is underexposed. Which of the following manipulations will produce diagnostically acceptable radiographs?

   A. Overdevelopment.
   B. Sight-development.
   C. Treatment with Farmer's Reducing Agent.
   D. None of the above.

27. D

28. In the chemistry of processing, potassium bromide:

   A. Is an activator for reducing agents.
   B. Is an activator for clearing agents.
   C. Is a component of the developing solution.
   D. Tends to increase radiographic fog.

28. C

29. The latent image consists of the accumulation of:

   A. Electrons in exposed silver bromide crystals.
   B. Atomic silver at the sensitization specks.
   C. Atomic silver in gelatin molecules.
   D. Electrons in photoconductance bands.

29. B

30. Which of the following can be used to reduce radiographic density?

   A. Sodium sulfite and hyposulfite.
   B. Sodium sulfite and potassium ferricyanide.
   C. Potassium bromide and potassium ferricyanide.
   D. Sodium thiosulfate and potassium ferricyanide.
   E. X rays and duplicating film.

30. D

31. Sodium sulfite is a component of:

   A. Developing solution.
   B. Fixing solution.
   C. A and B.
   D. None of the above.

31. C

32. Which of the following requires an acid pH for proper functioning?

   A. Sodium thiosulfate.
   B. Potassium alum.
   C. Potassium bromide.
   D. Sodium sulfite.

32. **B**

33. Which of the following is a hardening agent in film processing?

   A. Acetic acid.
   B. Potassium bromide.
   C. Potassium alum.
   D. Potassium hydroxide.

33. **C**

SECTION 12

THE DARKROOM, AUTOMATIC PROCESSING, AND FILM VIEWING

THE DARKROOM

The main function of a darkroom is to provide an environment where x-ray films can be handled and processed to provide an image of maximum diagnostic quality. To achieve this goal, the darkroom must be properly designed and equipped and must be manned by well-trained and conscientious personnel.

Let us first discuss design and equipment. Remember that the emulsion is sensitive not only to x rays, but also to (1) _____ and (2) _____, which are other forms of (3) _____ energy. The two prime sources of undesirable light in the darkroom are (4)_____ _____ and (5) _____.
If either of these is suspected, a simple procedure can be performed to check for undesirable light: (6) _____ _____.

Regardless of the source, the effect of undesirable light on x-ray film is (7) _____.

For Kodak* filters, be sure that you are familiar with the information contained in Table 12–1. Remember, however, that there are several film types that require a 7½ watt bulb; therefore, reading the manufacturer's instructions is important. Also, if two or more safelights are placed too close together but are at the correct distance from the working surface, (8) _____ of light may overlap, which can fog the film.

The importance of time-temperature processing has already been mentioned. The two most important pieces of equipment that will maintain the solutions at a constant temperature are the (9) _____ and the (10) _____.

---

*Eastman Kodak Co., Rochester, New York 14650.

1. light
2. heat
3. radiant
4. an "unsafe" safe-light
5. light leaks from outside the door
6. Remove an unexposed film from the packet. Place a paper clip on the film, and leave it in the vicinity of a suspected light leak for one or two minutes. The most common areas are at the edges of the door and under the safelight. Process the film. If the image of the paper clip shows up, the film has been exposed to undesirable light.
7. fog
8. undesirable areas
9. automatic temperature control
10. water-pressure control valve

TABLE 12–1. DARKROOM FILTERS

Filter Type	Size of Light Bulb (watts)	Use	Minimum Distance Above Countertop (feet)
ML-2	15	Intraoral film	4
6B	15	Extraoral film	4
GBX	15	All film types, including rare-earth screen film	4

The thermometer should be placed in the (11) _____, and an accurate timer should be on hand. Additionally, a (12) _____ chart should be within easy view from the processing station. Also, separate stirring paddles should be provided for the (13) _____ and the (14) _____ and should be used every day before (15) _____.

11. developer

12. time-temperature

13. developer
14. fixer
15. processing the first film

As far as handling the film is concerned, neatness and careful attention to the job at hand is the best way to proceed. In Table 12–2, try to identify the cause of each film-handling or processing error by covering the right column.

To avoid some of these common errors, remember these tips:

1. Use the (16) _____ chart.

16. time-temperature

TABLE 12–2. FILM-HANDLING AND PROCESSING ERRORS

Error	Cause(s)
Film fogged	Undesirable light
Brown spots on countertops, walls, clothing	Developer stain
White spots on countertops and walls	Fixer stain
Radiolucent spots on film	Developer artifact (film contaminated prior to processing)
Radiopaque spots on film	Fixer artifact (film contaminated prior to processing)
	Air bubble (inadequate agitation)
Film too dark (dense)	Overdeveloped (temperature too hot for selected time; selected time too long at a given temperature)
Film too light	Underdeveloped (inadequate attention to time-temperature charts)
Black lightninglike streaks	Inadequate humidity of air in darkroom (static electricity)
Black streaks beginning at clip marks	Film rack contaminated with developer
Black, grease pencil–like lines running horizontally across the film	Roller marks made by automatic processors
Half-moon or crescent-shaped black marks	Fingernail artifact
Black fingerprint	Finger contaminated with fluoride
Radiopaque line	Scratched emulsion
Top film(s) on rack un-processed or partially processed	Level of solution in tank too low
Processed film greenish, image poorly visible	Inadequate fixing
Sharply demarcated area of the film that is markedly lighter	One film stuck to another in the developing solution (owing to surface tension, only one side of the emulsion was processed; this area is therefore lighter)

2. The countertops should be (17) _____.

3. Hold the film by the (18) _____ between the (19) _____ and (20) _____ finger so that you do not touch the emulsion.

4. Film racks should be free of (21) _____ and (22) _____ contamination and should have some means of identifying (23) _____.

5. Do not overcrowd the (24) _____, as this results in errors and loss of films.

6. Things to check: (25) _____ strength, undesirable (26) _____, and (27) _____ _____ temperature.

7. The safelight should be at least (28) _____ feet above the countertop.

8. In most dental offices the fixer solution will last (29) _____ times as long as the developer solution.

9. The best darkroom in the world manned by the most competent personnel cannot make up for poor (30) _____ _____.

10. Having to repeat a film, for whatever reason, (31) _____ the radiation dose to the patient and (32) _____ the cost to the practitioner.

17.	clean
18.	edges
19.	thumb
20.	index
21.	developer
22.	fixer
23.	the patient
24.	processing tanks
25.	developer
26.	light leaks
27.	developer
28.	4
29.	two
30.	clinical exposure technique
31.	doubles
32.	doubles

AUTOMATIC PROCESSING

Identification of the Component Parts

Look at Figure 12–1 and see if you can identify the component parts of the typical automatic processor. Note that we have added the daylight-loader unit and the solution replenisher assembly. These may be optional for some units.

33. _____
34. _____
35. _____

33.	safety filter top
34.	developer solution
35.	roller film trans- porter

Automatic Dental X-Ray Film Processor

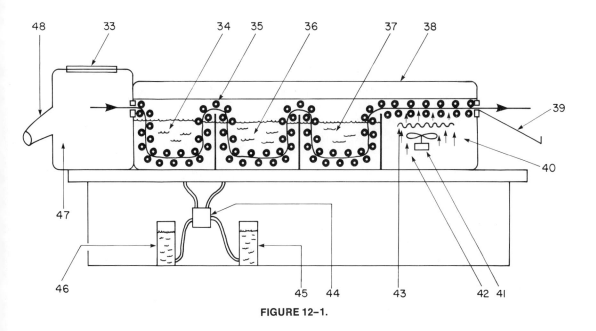

FIGURE 12-1.

36. _____	36. fixer solution
37. _____	37. water
38. _____	38. processor housing
39. _____	39. film-recovery slot or tray
40. _____	40. air flow
41. _____	41. air fan
42. _____	42. dryer unit
43. _____	43. dryer heater or heating element
44. _____	44. replenisher pump assembly (optional)
45. _____	45. fixer solution
46. _____	46. developer solution
47. _____	47. daylight-loader unit (optional)
48. _____	48. access opening or sleeve

Now that you know the parts of a typical automatic processor, look at Figure 12–2 and see if you can explain what happens to a film from the time it is loaded into the machine until the dry, processed film is delivered.

The exposed x-ray film is hand-stripped and inserted into the (49) _____ slot. This is normally done inside the

49. film feed

Automatic Dental X-Ray Film Processor

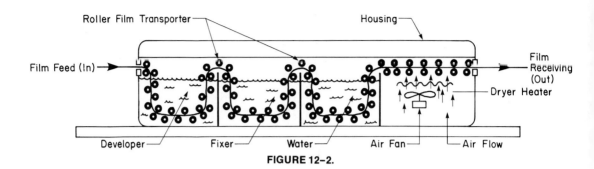

FIGURE 12–2.

darkroom; however, the processor may be located outside the darkroom if it is equipped with a (50) _____ loader. The film is pulled into the processor by the rolling motion of the (51) _____. It is rapidly transported through the following four stages:

1. The first stage consists of the (52) _____.
   This solution is superheated to approximately (53) _____, depending on the brand of machine used. The rollers transport the film down through the solution. The action of the rollers produces a constant squeegeeing of the film. This action, along with the forward movement of the film, causes the emulsion (54) _____ _____. This squeegeeing action also (55) _____ most of the developer solution from the (56) _____ before the film enters the next stage and (57) _____ the developer solution.

2. Next, the film is transported to the (58) _____.
   During this stage, the film is rapidly (59) _____ and (60) _____. As the rollers carry the film out of the fixer solution, the (61) _____ action of the rollers removes most of the fixer solution.

3. The film is then transported to the (62) _____.
   This stage consists of either a constant (63) _____ or a tank containing circulating (64) _____ and an overflow drain.

4. The last stage consists of the (65) _____. This is a constant blast of (66) _____ air.

---

50. **daylight**

51. **roller transport system**

52. **developer**

53. **80 to 95°F**

54. **to come in contact with fresh solution as the film advances through the developer**

55. **removes**
56. **emulsion**
57. **agitates**
58. **fixer**
59. **cleared (fixed)**
60. **hardened**
61. **squeegeeing**

62. **wash**
63. **spray**
64. **fresh water**

65. **dryer**
66. **heated, dry**

The (67) _____ action of the rollers dries the film further as it advances through the transport assembly.

5. After the drying stage, the processed film emerges from the unit at the (68) _____. This entire procedure should take approximately (69) _____ minutes. The flow time and temperature on most automatic processors can be adjusted by a (70) _____ and a (71) _____ _____.

67. squeegeeing

68. film-recovery slot or tray
69. 2.5 to 5
70. speed control
71. solution heater thermostat control

A problem guide (Table 12–3) follows, which discusses common processing problems. Please read it carefully and familiarize yourself with the correct procedures.

TABLE 12–3. PROBLEM GUIDE*

Problem	Cause	Correction
Film Surface Marks		
Pressure marks	Foreign material on roller	Clean rollers
	Rough handling of film before processing	Owing to sensitivity of film emulsions, gentle handling is needed
Film has greenish yellow hue	Depleted fixer	Replace fixer
	Improper film	Use film made for automatic processing
	Wrong fixer	Use rapid-process fixer
	Processor speed too fast	Reduce processor speed
Emulsion peeling	Deposits on developer roller	Clean roller
	Solution temperature too high	Turn off standby switch; check thermostat
	Wash water temperature too high	Reduce wash water temperature
	Improper film	Use film made for automatic processing
Film scratches	Rough handling of film before processing	Gentle handling of films is needed
	Sticking roller	Check racks, gears, and gear mesh
	Foreign material on roller	Clean rollers
	Burr on input slot	Remove burr
White chalky film	Lack of wash water	Check water supply
	Fixer precipitated	Replace fixer
Film Drying Problems		
Films damp or wet	Processing speed too fast	Increase processing time
	Defective dryer fan/heater	Replace defective fan/heater
	Improper film	Use film made for automatic processing
	Wrong developer and/or fixer	Use only rapid-process developer and fixer

TABLE 12–3. PROBLEM GUIDE (Continued)*

Problem	Cause	Correction
Film Density Problems		
Light films	Developer nearing exhaustion	Drain developer solution, clean tank, and fill with new developer solution
	Developer contaminated	Same as above
	Developer temperature too low	Turn on standby switch; plug in heater pad; check for defective thermostat or heating pad
	Processing speed too fast	Increase total processing time
	Exposure time too short	Increase exposure time in 20% increments
Dark films	Exposure time too long	Decrease exposure time in 20% increments
	Fixer in developer	Change developer
	Thermostat failure causing solutions to overheat	Replace thermostat
Fogged film	Incorrect safelight filter or bulb	Use a 6B filter with 15 watt bulb
	Excessive light	Check that safelight bulb is of proper wattage; check for light leaks in darkroom
	Developer temperature too high	Check thermostat; adjust or replace
	Light leak between processor and daylight loader	Block light leak with black tape
Gray films	No water in wash section	Add water

*Courtesy of Dr. Peter A. Fortier, New Orleans, Louisiana.

Types of Solutions Used

Several brands are available that produce excellent quality processing. Be certain that the solutions are labelled for (72) _____ processing use. This will ensure maximum life at 80 to 95°F. Additionally, these solutions are formulated with a hardener, which begins to act during the (73) _____ stage. This prevents (74) _____ _____.

72. **rapid or automatic**

73. **developing**
74. **sticking of the films in the roller transport system**

Replenishing

Replenishing is always carried out in proportion to the number of films processed. This procedure maintains adequate concentrations of chemicals, which ensures (75) _____ results between chemical changes. As a routine, the developer

75. **uniform**

126

and fixer tanks should be replenished (76) _____.
The best time of day to do this is in the (77) _____.
For high volume, replenishing may be repeated at (78) _____ to ensure uniform results throughout the day. Automatic replenishers are available and are preferred for (79) _____ and (80) _____ films.

76. **daily**
77. **morning**
78. **noon**

79. **high volume**
80. **extraoral**

Maintenance

All automatic processors will produce excellent results provided that an (81) _____ is instituted. This program should be posted near the machine and should include the following:

81. **effective mainten- ance program**

1. A (82) _____ time schedule for regular maintenance.

82. **routine**

2. The (83) _____ of the person who performed the maintenance.

83. **name**

3. Daily start-up and shut-down (84) _____.

84. **procedures**

4. Proper (85) _____ settings (set-up and adjustments).

85. **temperature and speed**

5. Solution levels and (86) _____ procedures.

86. **replenishment**

6. Instructions for (87) _____ all parts.

87. **cleaning**

Remember that the most important aspect of automatic processing is to be familiar with the (88) _____ _____. These should be reviewed on a regular basis, and all personnel who operate or maintain the equipment should be made fully aware of the importance of this step.

88. **manufacturer's instructions**

X-Ray Checker.* The purpose of an x-ray checker is to check for a malfunctioning x-ray machine or exhausted or contaminated developing solutions. To make an x-ray checker, you need one piece of cardboard, five layers of lead from the back of a periapical film, and adhesive tape.

_____
*Courtesy of Dr. Peter A. Fortier, New Orleans, Louisiana.

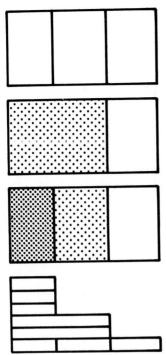

FIGURE 12–3. X-ray checker. (Courtesy of Dr. Peter A. Fortier, New Orleans, Louisiana.)

To construct the checker (see Fig. 12–3):

1. Divide the cardboard into thirds.
2. Cover two-thirds of the cardboard with two pieces of lead and tape it down.
3. Cover the last third with three or more pieces of lead (the first third is left uncovered).

Now you have an instrument that can check the quality of your x-ray machine and your developing solutions.

To use the checker:

1. Place your checker on top of a film and take an x ray using the same exposure settings used in the molar view for patients.
2. Develop the film in fresh developer and fixer. Repeat the first step several times, making six or eight films for future testing. Do not develop.
3. When the quality of your x-ray film is poor, develop one of the films you took in #2. Develop it in the solution you used for the questionable x-ray film.
4. If it is as good as the one you took on the first day, then the solutions are good and your x-ray machine should be further investigated. If it is of poor quality, then your solution is bad.
5. If the problem is a malfunctioning x-ray machine, take an x ray with the checker and develop it.

To avoid errors with automatic processors, remember these simple rules:

1. Maintain clean solutions and equipment (this is most important).
2. Replenish solutions often, depending on the use.
3. Maintain developing section at 80 to 95°F.
4. Do not put bent film in processor.
5. Do not feed film into processor too rapidly.
6. Keep transport sections in proper alignment.
7. Keep oil and grease off rollers.
8. Do not contaminate solutions.
9. Keep films straight when feeding into processor.
10. Initiate a maintenance program with careful attention to the details in the manufacturer's instructions.

VIEWING RADIOGRAPHS

Remember these five rules when viewing radiographs:

1. Radiographs should be viewed in a (89) _____ area with (90) _____ lighting.

89. quiet
90. subdued

2. The viewbox should have (91) _____ lighting. A (92) _____-intensity viewbox is ideal.

91. uniform
92. variable

3. All extraneous light should be (93) _____ (use cardboard to mask out the light around the mount).

93. blocked out

4. Use a good (94) _____ glass.

94. magnifying

5. Restrict the (95) _____ of the viewing field.

95. size

Sample Examination Questions

1. Which of the following safelight filters is recommended for developing screen-type films such as panoramic films?

   A. Kodak Morlite filter.
   B. Rinn Extra lite filter.
   C. Wratton series 6B filter.
   D. None of the above.

2. The safety of a darkroom safelight depends on the:

   A. Distance of the safelight from the work bench.
   B. Time the films are exposed to the safelight.
   C. Wattage of the bulb in the safelight.
   D. Speed of the film.
   E. All of the above.

3. The safety of safelight illumination does NOT depend on which of the following?

   A. Size of the darkroom.
   B. Wattage of the light bulb.
   C. Distance of the safelight from the workbench.
   D. Duration of time the film was exposed to the safelight.

4. The many differences between automatic and manual processing include which of the following?

   A. Processing solutions.
   B. Solution chemistry.
   C. Solution concentration.
   D. Transport mechanism.
   E. All of the above.

5. Which of the following factors contribute to fog with a resultant degradation of film quality?

   (1) Unsafe safelight.
   (2) Unsafe storage following exposure.
   (3) Overdevelopment.
   (4) High temperature development with no change in processing time.
   (5) Outdated emulsion.
   (6) White light leaks in the darkroom.
   A. 1, 2, 3, and 4.
   B. 1, 3, 5, and 6.
   C. 1, 2, 3, 5, and 6.
   D. 1, 3, 4, 5, and 6.
   E. All of the above.

1.	C
2.	E
3.	A
4.	E
5.	E

6. During the processing of ultraspeed film in a private dental office, which of the following is the most important source of film fog?

    A. Secondary radiation to the dental operatory.
    B. Unsafe safelight.
    C. Developing solutions that are too cold.
    D. Excessive fixation.

6. B

7. What is the most common cause of automatic processor jamming?

    A. Using depleted solutions in the processor.
    B. Using high solution temperatures in the processor.
    C. Feeding bent films into the processor.
    D. Feeding large films into the processor.

7. C

8. Radiographic density varies inversely with the:

    A. Radiolucency of the object.
    B. Quantity of silver in the radiograph.
    C. Quantity of x-radiation exposing the film.
    D. Quantity of incident viewing light transmitted through the radiograph.

8. D

9. The area of least radiographic density in a radiograph:

    A. Could be called *radiolucency*.
    B. Represents the area most translucent to the incident viewing light.
    C. Contains the greatest quantity of metallic silver.
    D. Has a radiographic density value of approximately 2.0.
    E. None of the above.

9. B

SECTION 13

RADIATION BIOLOGY

It is interesting to note that ionizing radiation can cause malignant neoplasms, can diagnose these tumors, and can destroy them. X rays, as you know, are a source of ionizing radiation. Radiation has biologic effects on any person exposed to even the smallest amount. Radiobiology is the study of the effects of ionizing radiation on biologic tissue. These effects are measurable and predictable, and their harmfulness is determined by a number of parameters. The National Council on Radiation Protection and Measurements uses these parameters to determine radiation protection criteria for various groups within the population.

The use of x rays for diagnostic purposes is part of the everyday life of dentists, dental hygienists, dental assistants, and other members of the dental team. We have a responsibility to ourselves and our progeny as well as our patients and neighbors in the immediate vicinity of our x-ray equipment. To protect these individuals, there are certain rules concerning the use of ionizing radiation that we must remember.

At present, these rules are taught only when they change as a result of research advances. The parameters of safe radiation exposure have been decreasing steadily since 1925, with the latest decrement occurring in 1970. As professional standards solidify in response to popular concern about radiation, it is quite possible that periodic updating will be required.

Therefore, we must continue to apply these rules over a span of many decades. To do this we must maintain a "healthy" respect for the biologic effects of ionizing radiation. A basic understanding of radiobiology will help us to do this, and it is in this spirit that we include this most important section.

RADIATION BIOLOGY AS IT RELATES TO DENTISTRY

Relative to our patients, we are not as interested in whole-body effects as in the effects on small portions of the organism. These effects have been subdivided into (1) _____ and (2) _____ effects. We will see more of these later in the section. In our consideration of the patient, we will follow a photon of x-radiation from the time it penetrates the skin until all of its energy has been dissipated.

1. **somatic**
2. **genetic**

Whenever we take a radiograph of a patient, we, the operators of the equipment, can be exposed to ionizing radiation. We are thus classified as (3) _____ exposed persons; different criteria are used to establish (4) _____ exposure limits for us. As occupationally exposed radiation

3. **occupationally**
4. **safe**

workers, we are more interested in (5) _____-body, (6) _____-term, (7) _____-dose exposures to (8) _____ radiation.

In general dentistry, we are less concerned about the following areas of radiation biology: therapeutic effects of ionizing radiation in the treatment of malignant neoplasms; the effects of larger doses of x-radiation as used in medical radiology; whole-body exposure to acute doses as in an atomic blast or when working with radioactive materials; the effects of injected radioactive isotopes as used in cellular labelling techniques and nuclear medicine; and a number of other applications that are not of direct interest to the dentist. Naturally, these effects are of great interest to the dental radiologist and those workers in specialized areas of dentistry that deal with these problems. There are a few exceptions within some of the specialized areas, and these will be discussed later in this section.

EFFECTS OF X-RADIATION ON DENTAL PATIENTS

We have already studied the interaction of x rays with matter, so it is not surprising to find that the harmful effects of x-radiation on our patients are produced by some of these same mechanisms.

When a beam of x-ray (9) _____ passes into a patient's tissues, the energy of the beam is dissipated. The average photon energy range of the beam used in dentistry is (10) _____ keV (kiloelectron volt). As the tissue absorbs this energy, most of it is ultimately converted into (11) _____, which produces no biologic damage. However, some of the energy results in minute amounts of (12) _____, which is usually repairable.

9. **photons**

10. **25 to 45**

11. **heat**

12. **biologic damage**

Now, let us see how biologic damage is produced. As the beam of x-ray photons enters the skin, the first or (13) _____ interaction occurs by means of either the photoelectric effect or the Compton effect. In the case of the Compton effect, a photon of x-radiation collides with a tissue electron, such as an outer valence electron of water. This results in a high-speed (14) _____, which is set into motion, and a lower-energy (15) _____ photon, which may interact with other tissue electrons. In the case of a photoelectric effect, all the energy of the photon is converted into electronic kinetic energy. In either case, the high-speed electron that is set into motion will give off its energy by the following mechanisms: (16) _____, (17) _____

13. **primary**

14. **electron**

15. **scattered**

16. **ionization**
17. **excitation**

_____, and (18) _____.
Additionally, bremsstrahlung radiation and heat are generated. Therefore, as the high-speed electron follows a track through the tissue, it produces chemical changes, which cause biologic damage. After a primary Compton interaction, the remaining incident photon energy is (19) _____. This, along with the bremsstrahlung radiation, can produce a number of further interactions. In fact, about (20) _____ interactions would have to take place to totally convert a single incident photon into electron (21) _____.
(22) _____ is a measure of the energy released by the ionizing particle (high-speed electron) along its track in tissue. It is usually expressed in units of keV per micron of track length.

As LET increases, the biologic effect of radiation increases, since the amount of energy released per unit of track length is greater. As the electron moves along its track it (23) _____
_____. The electron loses energy by a number of interactions such as (24) _____ and (25) _____. Since slowly moving charged particles lose energy faster than rapidly moving ones, LET gradually increases along the particle track. Just before the electron comes to a complete stop there is a dramatic increase in the amount of energy transferred. This is called the (26) _____ (see Figure 13–1).

Before leaving the subject of tracks, remember that in dental radiation, the ionizing particles that move along their tracks in tissue are (27) _____. At each interaction the fast-moving electron will lose some of its energy and slow down, and the direction of the track will change. The path of electron tracks is described as (28) _____. Additionally, the primary ionizing electron can eject another electron along its track, which has enough energy to produce a

18. breaking of molecular bonds

19. scattered

20. 30

21. motion
22. linear energy transfer (LET)

23. decelerates
24. ionization
25. excitation

26. Bragg peak

27. electrons

28. tortuous

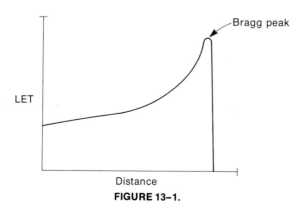

FIGURE 13–1.

track of its own. This energetic secondary electron's track or branch is known as a (29) _____ ray (see Figure 13–2). Delta rays transfer energy arising from the primary particle in areas outside or beyond the (30) _____ _____, thus increasing the area being affected.

The biologic effects of ionizing particles (e.g., fast-moving electrons) may be divided into (31) _____ and (32) _____ effects. Within cells, many molecular configurations or chemical compounds play a role in controlling biologic functions. These are designated as (33) _____ _____ for radiation. If the target is a complex molecule such as an enzyme, ionization or excitation might alter the molecule directly so that it is inactivated. This action of the radiation is called a (34) _____ effect.

The (35) _____ effects of ionizing radiation are a result of the production of (36) _____. These electronically excited chemical species, called (37) _____, have unpaired electrons and are therefore highly reactive. To achieve a chemically (38) _____ _____ state, these free radicals react with each other and their milieu. Thus, they may combine to form intracellular poisons such as (39) _____, or they may attack target molecules such as (40) _____ and (41) _____. These actions of ionizing radiation are known as (42) _____ effects.

29. delta
30. primary particle track

31. direct
32. indirect

33. targets

34. direct

35. indirect
36. free radicals

37. primary products

38. stable

39. hydrogen peroxide
40. DNA
41. RNA
42. indirect

Since water constitutes more than 70% of each cell, let us look at one interaction between water and ionizing radiation. When H_2O is irradiated, it may give rise to various reactive products:

$$H_2O \xrightarrow{\text{Radiation}} H_2O^* \rightarrow H\cdot + OH\cdot$$

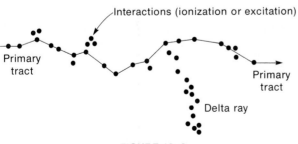

FIGURE 13–2.

Now the free radicals, having unpaired electrons, can react with each other to produce the following:

$$H \cdot + OH \cdot \ \rightarrow (43) \ \rule{2cm}{0.4pt}$$

$$H \cdot + H \cdot \ \ \rightarrow (44) \ \rule{2cm}{0.4pt}$$

$$OH \cdot + OH \cdot \rightarrow (45) \ \rule{2cm}{0.4pt}$$

The free radical can also react with (46) _____ , (47) _____ , (48) _____ , and (49) _____ . Indirect effects are much more important than direct effects in inducing biologic damage.

43. H_2O
44. H_2
45. H_2O_2 (hydrogen peroxide)
46. more water
47. its own reaction products
48. oxygen
49. organic molecules (indirect effects)

Generally, oxygen (50) _____ the effects of radiation on tissues. Oxygen reacts with the free radicals, thus producing further destructive chemical reactions with cell molecules. The biologic molecules that are believed to be most affected by radiation damage are the (51) _____ . DNA is contained within the (52) _____ of the cell. It consists of a double helix of two sugar phosphate chains and four bases: (53) _____ , (54) _____ , (55) _____ , and (56) _____ (see Figure 13–3).

50. enhances

51. nucleic acids

52. nucleus
53. adenine
54. guanine
55. cytosine
56. thymine

RNA is also found in the nucleus and is similar to DNA. RNA usually consists of one (57) _____ chain and contains three of the same bases as DNA; (58) _____ replaces thymine. Both DNA and RNA molecules must remain intact if a proper encoding phenomenon is to take place. Alterations in the DNA molecule will be reflected in altered messenger RNA; this will lead to defective (59) _____ synthesis at the (60) _____ , the sites of protein production in the (61) _____ .

57. sugar phosphate

58. uracil

59. protein
60. ribosomes
61. cytoplasm

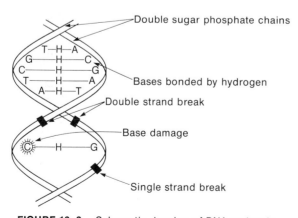

FIGURE 13–3. Schematic drawing of DNA molecule.

Four types of damage can occur to DNA and RNA: (62)_____ _____, (63) _____, (64) _____, and (65) _____. Evidence indicates that repair mechanisms probably exist for single strand breaks and some types of base damage, but (66) _____ are almost invariably lethal to the damaged cell.

The effects of ionizing radiation previously discussed affect the function of the cell in two ways: the direction of normal cell activities through enzymes and the genetic information for future generations. However, the number of cells affected by the radiation levels used in dentistry is very low. The probability of producing ionization, excitation, or the destruction of chemical bonds at significant levels is low. The action of repair mechanisms further reduces the probability of causing permanent damage. The occurrence of cell death has an even lower probability. Remember, however, that the effects of radiation are (67) _____. That is to say, with each exposure to radiation there is some (68) _____ followed by (69) _____. A small amount of unrepaired damage remains. This phenomenon is part of the reason why it is recommended that every possible precaution be taken to avoid overexposure of the patient and that a record be kept by the dentist in the patient's chart of each dose of radiation administered for (70) _____ purposes.

We are dealing here with statistics, and, while the probability is low, it cannot be denied that a finite probability of inducing biologic damage does exist when performing dental x-ray examinations. This risk includes the induction of leukemia, thyroid cancer, and cancer of the salivary glands.

At this point we should say a few words about dose-response relationships. Dose-response relationships are specific for the tissue irradiated and the type of radiation used. If the relationship is linear, the response of the tissue will be directly proportional to the dose. When presented graphically, this relationship appears as a (71) _____ line. Genetic damage and cancer induction are types of biologic damage currently believed to follow the linear pattern.

A nonlinear dose-response relationship is one in which the response is not proportional to the dose. When represented graphically, this relationship appears as a (72) _____ line. Very often these nonlinear relationships have a threshold, a dose level below which the effect does not occur. Examples of biologic damage following this type of dose-

62. **base damage (mainly cytosine, thymine, and uracil)**
63. **single chain breaks**
64. **double chain breaks**
65. **inactivation of DNA repair enzymes**
66. **double chain breaks**

67. **cumulative**

68. **damage**
69. **repair**

70. **diagnostic**

71. **straight**

72. **curved**

response relationship are the formation of cataracts and the production of erythema.

The only data available for estimating risks from low levels of ionizing radiation for human subjects have come from studies done on people who have received high levels of radiation, such as atomic bomb survivors or people who were accidentally overexposed for one reason or another. The figures from those data are extrapolated downward from these high radiation levels to much lower levels, using a dose-response relationship that describes the biologic effect under consideration. From these numbers it is then possible to estimate risk. As we have said, the risk is very low in dental radiography.

Summing up the effects on dental patients, White and Rose, in their 1979 *JADA* report of their research activities, concluded, "The risk from dental radiography, if it exists, is well within the range resulting from natural environmental levels of exposure"[1] (see Table 13–1).

Gonadal and Genetic Effects

For most of us, one of the points that was made during our dental education was that gonadal and fetal tissues are (73) _____ sensitive to ionizing radiation. It is for this reason that most of us use the (74) _____ to protect our patients and some sort of impenetrable (75) _____ to protect ourselves. The material that follows is included so that you may more fully understand this aspect of radiation biology, although it is much more applicable to medical uses of ionizing radiation (lower GI series, pelvic views, lumbosacral views, radiographs of the femur, and other radiographs such as the accumulation of injected radioactive nuclide in the bladder as used in nuclear medicine).

73. **very**
74. **leaded apron**

75. **barrier**

There is no reason in dentistry to directly expose the unprotected gonads or uterus of any patient. The fetus is most sensitive to radiation during the (76) _____ trimester, a period during which many women are uncertain or unaware of being pregnant. The one exception to this restriction might be in the detection of some ovarian teratomas, where (77) _____ structures are sometimes seen.

76. **first**

77. **toothlike**

When considering the effect of irradiation on the testes or ovaries, there are two main considerations: the somatic effects on these organs, and the (78) _____ effects on future progeny.

78. **genetic**

TABLE 13–1. RADIATION DOSES FROM DENTAL RADIOGRAPHY AND OTHER SOURCES

Source	Dose
Dental Radiography	
Dose to midcheek: molar periapical* (90 kVp; 8″ FFD)	885 mR
Dose to midcheek: molar periapical† (Film Speed D; 90 kVp; 8″ FFD)	983 mR
Dose to thyroid gland per intraoral film† (Film Speed D; 50 to 90 kVp; 8 to 16″ FFD)	2 to 4 mR
Dose to infraorbital region (approximates maximum possible values for lens of eye) per intraoral film† (Film Speed D; 50 to 90 kVp; 8 to 16″ FFD)	28 to 92 mR
Average cone tip exposure per single dental film‡ (average of all film speeds and exposure factors)	1138 mR
Average cone tip exposure per single dental film† (Film Speed D; 50 to 90 kVp; 8 to 16″ FFD)	175 to 570 mR
Estimated gonadal exposure per film in an 18-film full mouth survey†	0.04 mR
Estimated annual contribution to gonadal dose by dental x-rays§	0.01 to 0.15 mrem
Other Sources of Radiation	
Estimated annual contribution to gonadal dose by medical x-rays§	30 mrem
Maximum permissible exposure to the gonads, blood-forming organs, and lenses of the eyes per year for any individual‖	500 mrem
Estimated yearly per capita dose in year 2000 from all nuclear power plants and fuel reprocessing plants‖	0.4 mrem
Current yearly average exposure to radiation from natural sources# in:	
U.S. (overall)	130 mrad
Houston, Texas	60 mR
Denver, Colorado	200 mR
Espirito Santo, Brazil	3000 mR

*Bushong, S. C., et al.: Reduction of patient exposure during dental radiography. *Health Phys* 21:281, 1971.
†Alcox, R. W., Jameson, W. R.: Patient exposures from intraoral radiographic examinations. *JADA* 88:568–579, 1974.
‡*Population Exposure to X-Rays, US 1964*. Public Health Service Publication No. 1519. US Public Health Service, Oct. 1966.
§Report of the United Nations Scientific Committee on the effects of atomic radiations. General Assembly, Official Records, 17th Session Suppl. No. 16 (A/5216) New York, 1962.
‖National Council on Radiation Protection and Measurements Report No. 43. National Council on Radiation Protection and Measurements, 1975.
#Bushong, S. C.: Radiation exposure in our daily lives. *Physics Teacher* 15(3):135–144, 1977.

First, the somatic effects: The (79) _____ are the most radiosensitive cells of the germinal epithelium (see Appendix). Large doses of radiation may produce temporary or permanent (80) _____. Additionally, (81) _____ dysfunctions may occur. Irradiation of the gonads has a (82) _____ influence on the survival of the organism. Apart from the somatic effects previously mentioned, the (83) _____ effects are of prime importance. Remember that (84) _____ are made of DNA operons, which in turn make up a detectable gene; these are located within the (85) _____ of the sperm cell and ovum. A (86) _____ gene is one that has been altered in some way by the ionizing radiation and can give rise to abnormalities in the (87) _____. Although mutant genes attain a much (88) _____ degree of expression than normal genes, once formed they are highly stable and are inherited in the usual (89) _____ manner. It is for this reason that recessive traits inherited by the first generation may not be expressed for several (90) _____.

Ionizing radiation may produce a number of chromosomal aberrations. These aberrations may produce descendants with excessive, missing, or malformed parts. Such individuals are referred to as (91) _____. The aberrations may or may not be compatible with survival, and spontaneous miscarriages and stillbirths may occur.

The three most common chromosomal aberrations caused by ionizing radiation are: bodily removal of a part of a chromosome, known as (92) _____; a damaged section of a chromosome becoming attached to another chromosome, known as (93) _____; and a section of a chromosome becoming turned around with reference to its original configuration, known as (94) _____.

Generally, chromatid deletions are referred to as (95) _____ aberrations; they show a (96) _____ dose-response relationship and remain independent of (97) _____. On the other hand, chromatid exchanges show a (98) _____ dose-response relationship and are referred to as (99) _____ aberrations.

At this point, it should be noted that the gonads receive a very small amount of radiation in dental radiography. It has been estimated that the gonads receive less than 1/10,000 of the exposure delivered to the face. For a typical examination, this is comparable to the background radiation received by

79. **spermatogonia**

80. **sterility (infertility)**
81. **hormonal**
82. **negligible**

83. **genetic**
84. **chromosomes**

85. **nucleus**
86. **mutant**
87. **fetus**
88. **lower (most mutant genes are cytocidal, few survive)**

89. **mendelian**

90. **generations**

91. **aneuploids**

92. **deficiency**

93. **translocation**

94. **inversion**

95. **one-hit**
96. **linear**

97. **dose**
98. **nonlinear**
99. **two-hit**

each of us every day. This amount obviously can be reduced to virtually nil with the use of the protective apron.

As of this writing, we fully agree with White and Frey. In their 1977 paper they stated: "It may well be that risk to the United States population resulting from failure to obtain radiographs when indicated is considerably greater than the risk resulting from their use."[2]

Effects of Therapeutic Radiation Doses in the Area of the Oral Cavity

Therapeutic radiation doses is a term used to refer to the doses received by patients who have undergone radiation therapy, most often for the management of malignant neoplasms. The dose depends on the nature of the neoplasm, its location, and the total treatment plan including combined therapy with surgery and/or chemotherapy, hyperbaric oxygen, and other factors such as hyperthermia for melanomas. The average dose is approximately (100) _____ _____ rads, administered in 30 divided doses of (101) _____ rads each. When the oral epithelium is irradiated, the earliest detectable clinical change is (102) _____. This is usually followed by (103) _____ and desquamation of the surface layers. If the salivary glands are within the portal of irradiation, (104) _____ _____ begins after a period of (105) _____ week(s). The minor salivary glands are also affected and secrete approximately (106) _____% of the total volume of saliva. The most sensitive of the major salivary glands is the (107) _____ gland.

When the course of therapy has been completed and healing and recovery have occurred, (108) _____ may persist owing to permanent damage to the salivary glands. When this occurs, there is a danger of developing (109) _____ in the teeth, which may lead to (110) _____ when periapical inflammation develops as a result.

The oral mucosa usually remains more atrophic, with many (111) _____ vessels visible at its surface. When the jaws are within the portal of irradiation there is a danger of developing (112) _____. For this condition to occur, three factors must be present: (113) _____, (114) _____, and (115) _____. It is therefore imperative that all efforts be made to prevent the development of dental abscesses and the extraction of teeth and to avoid trauma from dental prostheses. Even after 20 years the danger of

100.	6000
101.	200
102.	erythema
103.	radiation mucositis
104.	xerostomia
105.	1
106.	50
107.	submaxillary
108.	xerostomia
109.	radiation caries
110.	osteoradionecrosis
111.	telangiectatic
112.	osteoradionecrosis
113.	radiation (therapeutic)
114.	trauma
115.	infection

developing osteoradionecrosis remains, especially in the (116) _____ because of (117) _____
_____ .

When the jaws of children are irradiated, tooth development may be (118) _____ . Once recovery has occurred, eruption of the irradiated teeth may (119) _____ .

The lens of the eye is highly susceptible to ionizing radiation. The most common sequela is (120) _____
_____ . However, the threshold dose for cataractogenesis is about (121) _____ , and the latent period is approximately (122) _____ years.

EFFECTS OF X-RADIATION ON DENTISTS, DENTAL HYGIENISTS, DENTAL ASSISTANTS, AND OTHER MEMBERS OF THE DENTAL TEAM

Except when we are patients, we (as members of the dental team) are most likely to be chronically exposed to (123) _____-dose, (124) _____-term x-radiation. Additionally, when proper radiation hygiene practices are not used, (125) _____ part of the body may be exposed any number of times.

Historically, dentists, such as Kells, eventually developed (126) _____ because they directly irradiated themselves each time they exposed a patient. Because of the unreliability of early x-ray tubes, the dentist would expose his own hand and view it in the (127) _____
to determine the correct exposure factors. Dentists and dental assistants used to hold the film in the patient's mouth or hold the cone or tube head to steady the machine. Because of the (128) _____ speed of the film, much (129) _____
_____ exposure times were used.

Today, members of the dental team understand that dental radiation can behave as a (130) _____ and can produce malignancies such as carcinoma of the finger. As a result, very few dental personnel willingly expose themselves directly to the beam.

116. mandible
117. damage to the vascular bed and lack of collateral blood supply
118. permanently arrested
119. be delayed (they usually erupt, but develop no further)

120. cataractogenesis and possible glaucoma
121. 250 rads
122. 10

123. low
124. long

125. any

126. carcinomas

127. fluoroscope

128. slow
129. longer

130. carcinogen

However, with inadequate protection at the timer switch, between operatories in group practices and large clinics, at the location of specialized equipment such as the cephalometric or panoramic machines, and in a variety of other situations, members of the dental team may be unknowingly exposed to (131) _____ doses of radiation.

The most important effects of such exposures are postulated to be a (132) _____ life span and a decrease in group vigor. Although these effects have been observed in animals with large doses of whole-body irradiation, such effects have not been observed in man. Though (133) _____ are known to have been induced in man, they are usually observed after a short-term exposure over the total body or most of it. Leukemia is also observed after external radiation in large amounts, rather than at low-dose rates over the total body. Therefore, the danger of developing (134) _____ may be less than it was once thought to be.

Finally, it has always been said that medical radiologists have a (135) _____ life expectancy than other medical doctors. Generally, studies such as that of Seltzer and Startwell have shown this to be true in the earlier days of medical radiology.[3] Since 1960 and the advent of modern radiation hygiene practices, no demonstrable life shortening has been detected.

MAXIMUM PERMISSIBLE DOSES

The National Council on Radiation Protection (NCRP) has published the following dose limits: The whole-body dose to all persons from background radiation is (136) _____ per year. As a person occupationally exposed to radiation, your annual dose limit is (137) _____. The annual dose of the general public is limited to (138) _____. Students may only be exposed to (139) _____ per year. In the Biological Effects of Atomic Radiation Report of 1956 it was estimated that the maximum permissible cumulative dose rate of man-made ionizing radiation per 30 years should not exceed (140) _____ of whole-body exposure.

To calculate the maximum permissible cumulative dose rate to the gonads, blood-forming organs, and lenses of the eyes for occupationally exposed persons over the age of 18, the following formula is used: (141) _____
_____.

All of the previously mentioned dose limits refer to the more sensitive tissues such as the gonads and red bone marrow. It

131. chronic low

132. shortened

133. leukemias

134. leukemia

135. shorter

136. 0.1 rem
137. 5 rems/year or 0.1 rem/week

138. 0.5 rem
139. 0.1 rem

140. 10 rems

141. $D = 5 \text{ rems} \times (N - 18)$, where D is tissue dose in rems and N is age in years

is interesting to note that for families of radioactive patients, individuals under 45 years are allowed (142) _____ per year, whereas individuals over 45 years are allowed (143) _____ per year. Greater detail on permissible doses may be found in the NCRP Report Number 43.[4]

142. **0.5 rem**

143. **5 rems**

In 1977, Stuart C. Bushong published the following data for radiologists and x-ray technicians in four Houston hospitals: The average diagnostic x-ray worker will receive about (144) _____ per year, whereas some personnel involved in cinefluorographic studies may routinely receive (145) _____ per year.[5] Interestingly, more than 70% of nuclear reactor personnel receive less than (146) _____ per year.

144. **500 mrem**

145. **3000 mrem**
146. **100 mrem**

You may have surmised by now that the survival or general well-being of the organism depends on the size of the dose and whether the dose was delivered to the whole body or only a portion of it. For example, a whole-body dose of (147) _____ is lethal to most humans, whereas a total of 6000 rads in divided doses to an enlarged lymph node in the neck of an individual with Hodgkin's disease will usually produce a cure or at least a remission of the disease and survival of the patient.

147. **400 rads**

It may be of some value to you to know some of the dosages to individuals who receive radiation from various diagnostic and background sources. The following tables are included for your reference and future use.

(NOTE: Owing to a wide variety of factors, the literature is highly inconsistent from one study to another for these values. It is recommended that the reader consult the quoted sources to evaluate the parameters from which the data were obtained.)

TABLE 13-2. RECOMMENDED MAXIMUM RADIATION EXPOSURES TO ENTRANCE SURFACE TISSUE*

Examination (projection)	Dose (mR)
Chest (PA)	30
Skull (Lateral)	300
Abdomen (AP)	750
Cervical Spine (AP)	250
Thoracic Spine (AP)	900
Full Spine (AP)	300
Lumbosacral Spine (AP)	1000
Retrograde pyelogram (AP)	900
Feet (DP)	270
Dental (Bite-wing or periapical)	700

*Carter, J. E.: Radiation protection guidance to federal agencies for diagnostic x-rays. Office of the Federal Register, February 1, 1978, vol. 43, No. 22.

TABLE 13-3. AVERAGE ENTRANCE SKIN DOSE AS ESTIMATED BY THE U.S. PUBLIC HEALTH SERVICE IN 1970

Type of Examination	Dose (mrad)
Chest	41
Skull	307
Abdomen	893
Cervical spine	223
Lumbosacral spine	2027
Intravenous pyelogram	549
Extremities	93
Cholecystography	577
Lumbar spine	1786
Upper GI fluoroscopy	660
Barium enema	1228

TABLE 13-4. DOSES TO BODY SITES DURING CEPHALOMETRY*†

Sites	Dose (mrads)
Lens of eye	23
Pituitary fossa	15
Thyroid gland	29
Skin	50
Maxillary sinus	22
Ethmoid sinus	27
Mandibular notch	22
Mandible angle	28
Mandible symphysis	11
Cervical spine	7

*120 kVp; 11.8 mAs; FFD 165 cm.
†From Antoku et al.: Doses to critical organs from dental radiography. Oral Surg 41(2):251-260, 1976.

TABLE 13-5. DOSES TO BODY SITES DURING PANTOMOGRAPHY*

Sites	Dose (mrad) Semens, Type OP-2† (Field: 1 × 15 cm)	Morita, Panex‡ (Field: 0.5 × 23 cm)
Lens	6	12
Pituitary fossa	27	28
Thyroid gland	269	38
Skin: molar	34	5
premolar	12	5
lip	9	2
posterior neck	187	12
Maxillary sinus	13	7
Ethmoid sinus	15	5
Mandibular notch	539	78
Mandible angle	111	60
Mandible symphysis	23	5
Cervical spine	150	19

*From Antoku et al.: Doses to critical organs from dental radiography. *Oral Surg* 41(2):251–260, 1976.
†85 kVp; FFD 50 cm; 12 seconds; 15 mA.
‡90 kVp; FFD 74 cm; 23 seconds; 3.5 to 13.5 mA.

TABLE 13-6. MEAN BONE MARROW DOSE (MREM) BY SITE IN MANDIBLE*

Site	Panorex	Panelipse	Orthopantomograph	Intraoral	Collimated Intraoral	Lateral Cephalometric
Right third molar	22.0	56.3	29.9	510	183	33.8
Right first molar	12.1	17.5	26.7	821	261	25.6
Right first premolar	9.02	16.7	20.2	1143	326	29.0
Symphysis	8.71	16.0	19.3	988	422	17.7
Left first premolar	9.13	20.1	18.2	1080	299	9.84
Left first molar	13.2	25.2	22.0	826	284	7.74
Left third molar	24.8	71.0	30.9	580	192	7.57
Mean	14.1	31.8	23.9	850	282	18.8

*From White, S. C., Rose, T. C.: Absorbed bone marrow dose in certain dental radiographic techniques. *JADA* 98(4):553–558, 1979.

TABLE 13-7. MEAN BONE MARROW DOSE (MREM) BY SITE IN CERVICAL SPINE*

Site	Panorex	Panelipse	Orthopantomograph	Intraoral	Collimated Intraoral	Lateral Cephalometric
C-2	19.2	30.4	68.1	205	37.5	14.1
C-6	7.03	17.0	38.3	27.6	10.7	16.1
Mean	13.1	23.7	53.2	116	24.1	15.1

*From White, S. C., Rose, T. C.: Absorbed bone marrow dose in certain dental radiographic techniques. *JADA* 98(4):553–558, 1979.

Sample Examination Questions

1. Bone:

    (1) Absorbs the same amount of radiation as soft tissue.
    (2) Transmits more radiation than soft tissue.
    (3) Absorbs more radiation than soft tissue.
    (4) Absorbs the same amount of radiation as water.

  A. 1.
  B. 3.
  C. 2 and 4.
  D. All of the above.
  E. None of the above.

        1. B

2. Cell sensitivity to radiation is more pronounced:

    (1) During mitosis.
    (2) During periods of increased metabolism.
    (3) During embryonic development.
    (4) In muscle cells.
    (5) In nerve cells.

  A. 1, 2, and 3.
  B. 1, 2, and 5.
  C. 1, 3, and 5.
  D. 2, 3, and 4.
  E. 2, 3, and 5.

        2. A

3. Which of the following tissues is most susceptible to radiation?

  A. Nerve tissue.
  B. Muscle tissue.
  C. Brain tissue.
  D. Blood-forming tissue.

        3. D

4. Which of the following is most radiosensitive?

  A. Young bone.
  B. Nerve.
  C. Muscle.
  D. Gonads.

        4. D

5. The theory that explains cellular damage by x rays is the:

    A. Direct action poison-chemical theory.
    B. Indirect action poison-chemical theory.
    C. Bremsstrahlung action theory.
    D. Indirect nonionizing theory.

5. B

6. The currently recognized official maximum permissible dose (MPD) of radiation to an occupationally exposed person is:

    A. 0.1 rem/week.
    B. 0.2 rem/week.
    C. 0.3 rem/week.
    D. 0.4 rem/week.
    E. 0.5 rem/week.

6. A

7. It is well documented that x rays react at the cellular level and can cause biologic damage. In Figure 13–4, a photon is shown interacting with one molecule of water, resulting in:

    A. Excitation.
    B. Electrolyte formation.
    C. Attenuation.
    D. Free radical formation.

7. D

8. Which of the following is NOT a critical factor in the radiation response of cells?

    A. Cellular differentiation.
    B. Size of cells.
    C. Metabolic activity.
    D. Mitotic rate.

8. B

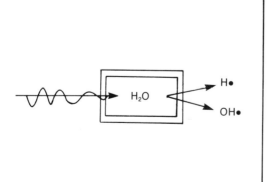

FIGURE 13–4.

9. Theoretically, the biologic response to a given dose of radiation would be greater (more severe) with:

    A. An anoxia of the tissue being irradiated.
    B. A higher dose rate.
    C. A smaller area of tissue exposure.
    D. Lower linear energy transfer (LET).

9. B

10. Which of the following x rays are most apt to be absorbed by the skin?

    A. Central x rays.
    B. Filtered x rays.
    C. Long-wavelength x rays.
    D. Short-wavelength x rays.

10. C

11. Which of the following latent effects can be associated with low-dose, whole-body radiation?

    A. Shock.
    B. Epistaxis.
    C. Epilation.
    D. Leukemia.

11. D

12. The latent period related to radiation biology is that period between:

    A. Exposure of the film and development of the images.
    B. Exposure to x-radiation and the appearance of clinical symptoms.
    C. The states of cell rest and cell mitosis.
    D. Subsequent doses of x-radiation.

12. B

13. On an average, the dose rate from natural background radiation is about:

    A. .5 mrem/year.
    B. 5 mrem/year.
    C. 60 mrem/year.
    D. 130 mrem/year.

13. D

14. The first clinically observable reaction to radiation overexposure is:

    A. Loss of hair.
    B. Reddening of the skin.

14. B

C. Loss of alimentary epithelium.
D. Agenesis of blood cells.

15. In therapeutic radiation, x rays are used to:

    A. Destroy tissue.
    B. Increase mitotic activity.
    C. Heat tissue.
    D. Dehydrate tissue.

16. A certain amount of radiation is needed before the clinical signs of damage to somatic cells appear. The amount of radiation after which damage can be produced is called the:

    A. Latent dose.
    B. Threshold dose.
    C. Hazard dose.
    D. Background radiation dose.
    E. Scattered radiation dose.

17. If you receive more than 100 mR in a week as a radiation worker, you should:

    A. Evaluate the radiation protection measures used in your dental office.
    B. Not work with radiation until you dissipate the 100 mR.
    C. Go on a vacation.
    D. Find another job.

18. As a radiation worker, you should not be exposed to more than 5 rem a year. But in x-raying yourself for dental treatment, you are exposed to about 5 rem. Which of the following reconciles these contradictory statements?

    A. Since you need dental radiographs, you can be given an unlimited amount of radiation.
    B. As a patient you can be given any amount of radiation, regardless of damage.
    C. Exceptions can be made.
    D. Whole-body radiation is different from specific-region radiation.

19. Generally, the most radiosensitive cells in an organism are those that:

    (1) Will undergo rapid mitosis.
    (2) Will undergo many mitoses.
    (3) Are the most primitive in their differentiation.
    (4) Are the most highly specialized.
A. 1 and 2.
B. 2 and 3.
C. 1, 2, and 3.
D. 2, 3, and 4.

19. C

20. If the dental hygienist or assistant holds the film in the patient's mouth for a prolonged period of time while making an x-ray exposures he or she may contract:

    (1) Tuberculosis.
    (2) Osteoradionecrosis.
    (3) Leukemia.
    (4) Carcinoma.
A. 1 and 2.
B. 2 and 3.
C. 2, 3, and 4.
D. All of the above.

20. C

21. Living tissue may develop which of the following after receiving damaging doses of x-radiation?

    (1) Regrowth of blood vessels.
    (2) Ulcer formation.
    (3) Epilation.
    (4) Increased hair growth.
    (5) Loss of bone.
A. 1, 3, and 5.
B. 2, 3, and 4.
C. 2, 3, and 5.
D. 2, 4, and 5.

21. C

22. Some examples of somatic cells in the human are:

    (1) Chromosomes.
    (2) Blood.
    (3) Muscles.
    (4) Genes.
    (5) Nerves.
A. 1, 2, and 4.
B. 1, 3, and 4.
C. 2, 3, and 4.
D. 2, 3, and 5.
E. 3, 4, and 5.

22. D

23. X-ray absorption is inversely related to the:

    A. Wavelength.
    B. Energy of the x-ray beam.
    C. Z number of the object exposed.
    D. Thickness of the object exposed.

24. The maximum permissible dose from diagnostic x rays for a patient in one year is:

    A. 500 mrem.
    B. 788 mrem.
    C. 5 rem.
    D. Not specified.

25. Which of the following effects is NOT considered dependent on dose rate?

    A. Death of the organism.
    B. Local somatic effects.
    C. Genetic effects.
    D. Fetal somatic effects.

26. The acute radiation syndrome:

    A. Invariably results in the death of the individual exposed.
    B. Could be induced in a sensitive individual with a radiation dose of 5 rem.
    C. Occurs when the head and neck area is exposed to a radiation dose of 400 to 500 rem.
    D. None of the above.

27. LD_{50} (30d) stands for the:

    A. Dose of radiation that leads to the death of 30 experimental animals when 50 are irradiated.
    B. Lethal dose to 25 out of 50 experimental animals within 30 days following an acute exposure.
    C. Lethal dose to 50% of the experimental animals with the dose fractionated over 30 days.
    D. Dose of radiation that kills 50% of a sample irradiated.

28. A radiation dose of 400 rem given locally to the arm would most likely cause:
    A. Erythema.
    B. Acute radiation syndrome.

23.	B
24.	D
25.	C
26.	D
27.	B
28.	A

C. Carcinoma of the skin.
D. Bone marrow death.

29. The highest incidence of radiation-induced anomaly production occurs:

    A. Immediately following conception.
    B. During organogenesis.
    C. In disease-complicated aging.
    D. When metabolism is reduced.

30. Which of the following is the earliest clinical symptom for an individual exposed to a mid-lethal radiation dose sufficient to cause acute radiation syndrome?

    A. Nausea and vomiting.
    B. Diarrhea.
    C. Loss of hair.
    D. General discomfort.
    E. Fever.

31. When an x-ray photon enters the skin, it sets in motion a high-speed tissue electron. This reaction is called the:

    A. Target theory.
    B. Threshold dose.
    C. Primary interaction.
    D. Recoil electron.

32. When a high-speed tissue electron is set in motion, it loses its energy by which of the following mechanisms?

    (1) Ionization.
    (2) Excitation.
    (3) Breaking of molecular bonds.
    (4) Heat generation.
    A. 4.
    B. 1, 2, and 3.
    C. 1, 2, and 4.
    D. All of the above.

33. The mechanisms by which an x-ray photon causes damage to tissues are:

    (1) Ionization.
    (2) Excitation.

        (3)   Breaking of molecular bonds.
        (4)   Bremsstrahlung.
        (5)   Scatter radiation.
        (6)   Delta-ray interactions.
        (7)   Heat generation.
    A.   1, 3, 4, 5, and 6.
    B.   1, 3, 4, 5, and 7.
    C.   1, 2, 3, 4, 5, and 6.
    D.   1, 3, 4, 5, 6, and 7.

34. About how many scattering interactions would be re-   34.   A
     quired to completely convert a single incident x-ray
     photon into electron motion?

     A.   30.
     B.   200.
     C.   300.
     D.   2000.

35. Which of the following is a unit of radiation absorbed   35.   D
     dose expressed in joules per kilogram of irradiated   1 gray = 1 Gy
     tissue?   = 1 J/kg
                                                                               = 100 rads
     A.   Roentgen (R).
     B.   Curie.
     C.   rem.
     D.   Gray (Gy).

36. The doubling dose is that dose: 36.   C

     A.   In which the LD_{50} is doubled.
     B.   In which the rads delivered are doubled.
     C.   That causes a doubling of gene mutation.
     D.   That causes a doubling of interactions along the
          track of a high-speed electron.

37. The delta ray is produced by: 37.   B

     A.   Interactions along a secondary track.
     B.   A fast-moving secondary electron moving away
          from the primary electron track.
     C.   The collision of a secondary electron with the
          primary track.
     D.   The collision of the incident photon with a secon-
          dary electron.

38. The Bragg peak is an abrupt increase in the LET:

    A. Just before the fast-moving electron comes to a stop.
    B. And involves a decrease in the energy transferred.
    C. Measured at any point along the primary track.
    D. And occurs at peak electron velocity.

38. A

39. Which of the following kinds of radiation-induced damage to the DNA molecule are considered repairable?

    (1) Single chain breaks.
    (2) Double chain breaks.
    (3) Base damage.
    (4) Inactivation of DNA repair enzymes.

    A. 1 and 3.
    B. 1, 2, and 3.
    C. 1, 3, and 4.
    D. All of the above.

39. A

40. RNA differs from DNA in that it consists of a single sugar phosphate chain and that its base uracil replaces:

    A. Thymine.
    B. Guanine.
    C. Cytosine.
    D. Adenine.

40. A

APPENDIX

Bergonie-Tribondeau Law

The radiosensitivity of living tissues varies as follows:
1. Mature cells are most resistant to radiation. Undifferentiated cells are highly radiosensitive.
2. Younger tissue and organs are more radiosensitive.
3. Radiosensitivity increases with metabolic activity.
4. Rapidly proliferating cells are more radiosensitive.

Cell Sensitivity (in decreasing order)

Highly Sensitive
1. Mature and immature lymphocytes
2. Spermatogonia
3. Intestinal epithelium
4. Differentiating oocytes and embryonic cells
5. Epithelium

Less Sensitive
1. Connective tissue
2. Muscle
3. Bone
4. Nerve

References

1. White, S. C., Rose, T. C.: Absorbed bone marrow dose in certain dental radiographic techniques. *JADA* 98(4):553–558, 1979.
2. White, S. C., Frey, N. W.: An estimation of somatic hazards to the United States population from dental radiography. *Oral Surg* 43(1):152–159, 1977.
3. Seltzer, R., Startwell, P. E.: The influence of occupational exposure to radiation on the mortality of American radiologists and other medical specialists. *Am J Epidemiol* 81(2):1965.
4. National Council on Radiation Protection and Measurements Report No. 43. National Council on Radiation Protection and Measurements, 1975.
5. Bushong, S. C.: Radiation exposure in our daily lives. *Physics Teacher* 15(3):135–144, 1977.
6. Alcox, R. W.: Biological effects and radiation protection in the dental office. *Dent Clin North Am* 22(3):517–532, 1978.
7. Bengtsson, G.: Maxillo-facial aspects of radiation protection, focused on recent research regarding critical organs. *Dentomaxillo Facial Radiol* 7:5–14, 1978.

SECTION 14

RADIATION SAFETY
AND PROTECTION

Now that we have studied some of the major effects of ionizing radiation on biologic tissues, it is important that we protect ourselves and our patients from any possible deleterious effects. Before studying this in some detail, there are several considerations with which you should be familiar.

(1) _____ refers to the direct radiation emanating from the cone of the x-ray machine and is often referred to as the "useful beam."

1. **primary radiation**

(2) _____ refers to radiation emitted by any matter that is being irradiated by x rays. (3) _____ _____ radiation is a form of secondary radiation and emanates mainly from the soft tissues of the patient's face and the pointed plastic cone.

2. **secondary radiation**
3. **scattered**

(4) _____ refers to all radiation emanating from the x-ray machine with the exception of the primary beam.

4. **leakage radiation**

National Council on Radiation Protection Report No. 35 makes several rulings about radiation safety. For intraoral radiography, the useful beam shall be restricted to a diameter of not more than (5) _____ at the end of the cone. Currently, most open-ended cones have a diameter of 2.75 inches. The x-ray timer should permit making reproducible radiographs with exposures as short as (6) _____ second. The aluminum equivalents of the total filtration in the useful beam should not be less than those listed in Table 14–1.

5. **3 inches**

6. **1/60**

TABLE 14–1. ALUMINUM EQUIVALENTS OF TOTAL FILTRATION DURING PRIMARY RADIATION

Operating Potential	Minimum Total Filtration (Inherent + Added)
< 50 kVp	(7) _____ mm Al
50 to 70 kVp	(8) _____ mm Al
> 70 kVp	(9) _____ mm Al

7. **0.5**
8. **1.5**
9. **2.5**

The purpose of filtration is to absorb the low frequency–long wavelength x rays that form a part of the heterogeneous beam emanating from the focal spot. This component of the x-ray beam should be (10) _____ for several reasons: it has a (11) _____ penetrating ability; it is a source of (12) _____ to the patient; it is of (13) _____ diagnostic value; and it is a source of (14) _____ on the exposed radiograph. The filter should be located as (15) _____ to the window of the tube housing as possible.

Selective filtration is being used more often to optimize the spectral characteristics of the x-ray beam. Radiation that is too "soft" is almost totally absorbed in the patient's tissues, thus giving the patient an unnecessary dose. On the other hand, radiation that is too "hard" is inefficiently absorbed by the film emulsion. Higher energies produce lower contrast films, whereas lower energies are so completely absorbed that inferior (high contrast ratio) radiographs result. The energy of dental x rays is in the 25 to 50 keV range because differences in tissue absorption are detectable at the film plane with a minimum absorbed dose to the patient.

PROTECTION OF THE PATIENT

Generally, the routine, daily application of these simple rules will minimize exposure of the patient to ionizing radiation:

1. Always shield the patient with a (16) _____ _____ when taking x rays. The most important organs to shield are the (17) _____ _____.

2. (18) _____ the beam to the smallest size that will yield consistent quality radiographs. For most periapical and bite-wing films, the (19) _____ cone and the (20) _____ beam-positioning and collimating device are most effective.

3. Never use more (21) _____ than is required for a properly exposed radiograph. Use (22) _____ film and intensifying (23) _____ and pay close attention to the (24) _____ recommended by the manufacturer of the film. Good clinical and darkroom technique is most important to minimize (25) _____. Additionally, the use of (26) _____ film packets and (27) _____ films is encouraged when two or more sets of films are required.

10. eliminated
11. poor, low
12. increased radiation
13. no
14. fog
15. close

16. leaded apron with a thyroid extension
17. gonads and thyroid

18. collimate

19. rectangular
20. rectangular

21. radiation
22. fast
23. screens
24. exposure values

25. retakes
26. double
27. duplicate

Copying X-Ray Films

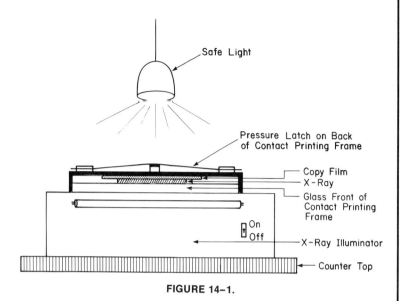

FIGURE 14–1.

Any radiograph may be duplicated by simply placing the film to be copied on top of a piece of unexposed copy film. Place the two films inside any standard contact printing frame, with the film to be copied outermost against the glass. Place the contact printer on top of a view box. Turn the view box on for approximately 3 seconds, and turn it off. (This, of course, is carried out in the darkroom.) Process the copy film in the usual manner, either with wet tanks or through the automatic processor. Several film-copying machines are available commercially.

4. When a processed film is too dark or dense because of overdevelopment or overexposure, lighten the image with (28) _____. This consists of one part (29) _____ and one part (30) _____. Agitate the film in this solution until the film is light enough to interpret. If the film is usable, a (31) _____ has been avoided.

28. **Farmer's Reducing Agent (available commercially)**
29. **potassium thiosulfate**
30. **potassium ferricyanide**
31. **retake**

5. The dental office or institution should have a quality assurance program. A (32) _____ program ensures diagnostic excellence through the routine monitoring of equipment and personnel. The use of a (33) _____ will verify the accuracy of the mA, kVp, and timer. Additionally, the (34) _____ will serve as an easy check for deterioration of processing solutions.

32. **quality assurance**
33. **step wedge, a Wisconsin test cassette, and a spinning top**
34. **sensitometer**

6. Avoid retakes; each one (35) _____ the dose of radiation to the patient.

35. **doubles**

PROTECTION OF THE OPERATOR AND STAFF

1. Use (36) _____-lined walls or the equivalent (concrete, brick, or sheetrock). Unpublished research has shown that four layers of half-inch sheetrock are sufficient to line the walls of rooms where dental x-ray equipment is used.

36. **lead**

2. The operator should never hold the (37) _____ or the (38) _____ when x rays are being taken.

37. **film**
38. **tube head**

3. The operator should stand at least (39) _____ feet away from the (40) _____ when radiographs are being exposed.

39. **6**
40. **tube head, source**

4. When exposing radiographs, the operator should always stand behind a (41) _____ that is impenetrable by x rays. If he needs to see the patient during the procedure, he may look at the patient through a (42) _____ glass aperture.

41. **barrier**

42. **leaded**

5. The operator should never stand directly in front of or (43) _____ the path of the primary beam. The safest position for most intraoral radiographs is (44) _____ degrees away from the tube head and behind the patient.

43. **directly behind**

44. **90 to 135**

6. Operators should subscribe to a (45) _____ monitoring service to be certain that they have not been exposed to any undue amounts of radiation. All users of x-ray equipment should have a (46) _____ record for each patient.

45. **personnel**

46. **radiation history**

7. All owners and operators of x-ray equipment should cooperate with federal and state officials and agencies in the matter of routine safety checks and personnel monitoring. Adherence to radiation protection regulations and equipment modifications is to be greatly encouraged.

Sample Examination Questions

1. Depending on the circumstances, when films are to be held in the mouth of a child, the dental radiologist should:

    (1) Hold them himself.
    (2) Ask the assistant to hold the film.
    (3) Ask a parent or guardian to hold the film.
    (4) Use film holders.
  A. 1 and 4.
  B. 2 and 3.
  C. 2 and 4.
  D. 3 and 4.

                1. D

2. For dental radiography, the recommended collimation of the radiation beam of the cone tip at the patient's skin surface is:

  A. 2.75 inches.
  B. 3 inches.
  C. 4 inches.
  D. 5 inches.

                2. B

3. A dentist is using a film badge service to measure his radiation exposure. The service reports that the badge was exposed to 500 millirems in the previous month. The dentist should:

  A. Stop taking x-ray films immediately.
  B. Report to a physician for a blood count.
  C. Ignore the report because the reading is insignificant.
  D. Evaluate his x-ray procedures and take steps to reduce unnecessary radiation.

                3. D

4. A pregnant woman:

  A. Should be advised of her legal rights before being irradiated.
  B. Should be warned about possible miscarriage.
  C. Should never be irradiated for dental radiographs.
  D. May be irradiated for dental radiographs by taking the necessary precautions.

                4. D

5. In normal dental diagnostic procedures, the principal hazard to the operator is produced by:

   A. Gamma radiation.
   B. Primary radiation.
   C. Secondary radiation.
   D. None of the above.

5. C

6. Film badge dosimetry is:

   A. A process that uses film that is sensitive to x, beta, and gamma rays.
   B. Not important to use in modern times.
   C. Only useful if occlusal films are exposed.
   D. Not sensitive to gamma rays.

6. A

7. Which of the following is mandatory in radiation protection for the patient?

   A. Gonadal shields.
   B. High-speed film.
   C. Collimator.
   D. Use of long, open-ended, lead-lined cones.

7. C

8. Which of the following is least effective in reducing patient radiation dose?

   A. Fast films.
   B. Higher kilovoltage.
   C. Proper collimation.
   D. Increased filtration.

8. B

9. The operator should NOT hold the:

   A. Film during exposure.
   B. Tube during exposure.
   C. Patient during exposure.
   D. All of the above.

9. D

10. Lead aprons are used:

   A. Only on pregnant women.
   B. To reassure patients.
   C. To reduce scatter to the film.
   D. On all patients.

10. D

11. Figure 14–2 illustrates the x-ray tube head from above with the central ray located as shown. During exposure of x rays, the safest operator position is at:

    (1) 3.
    (2) 2 or 4.
    (3) Halfway between 2 and 3.
    (4) Halfway between 3 and 4.
A. 1.
B. 2.
C. 1 and 2.
D. 3 and 4.

11. D

12. Secondary radiation is:

    (1) Less when kVp is increased.
    (2) Most detrimental to the patient.
    (3) Less deeply penetrating than primary radiation.
    (4) Proportional to the square of the distance the operator stands from the patient.
A. 1, 2, and 3.
B. 1, 3, and 4.
C. 2, 3, and 4.
D. All of the above.

12. C

13. The chief hazards to the operator in roentgenographic work are:

    (1) Exposure to the radiation coming directly from the x-ray cones.

13. D

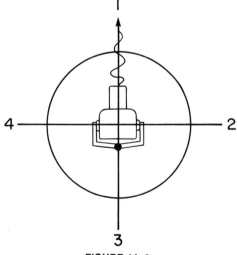

FIGURE 14–2.

    (2) Exposure to tube-head leakage.

    (3) Exposure to secondary radiation emitted from the patient during an exposure.

    (4) Radiation coming from an adjacent room.

A. 1, 2, and 3.

B. 1, 3, and 4.

C. 2, 3, and 4.

D. All of the above.

14. Some of the most effective means of controlling secondary radiation are:

    (1) Shielding.

    (2) Increasing kVp.

    (3) Using filters.

    (4) Decreasing film speed.

A. 1 and 3.

B. 2 and 3.

C. 1, 2, and 3.

D. 2, 3, and 4.

14. A

SECTION 15

HISTORICAL NOTES

It is universally known that (1) _____ _____ is credited with the discovery of the x ray in the year (2) _____ in Wurzberg, Bavaria. The first radiograph consisted of an image of the hand of Roentgen's wife, (3) _____. The exposure time using the Hittorf-Crookes tube was (4) _____ minutes. For his work, Roentgen received the (5) _____ Prize in the year (6) _____.

1. **Wilhelm Conrad Roentgen**
2. **1895**

3. **Bertha**
4. **15**
5. **Nobel**
6. **1901**

Only 14 days after Roentgen announced his amazing discovery, (7) _____ of Braunschweig, Germany made the first dental radiograph. His exposure time was 25 minutes.

7. **Dr. Otto Walkhoff**

The first intraoral radiographs were made in the year (8) _____. Although Dr. (9) _____ of New Orleans is generally credited with having taken the first intraoral radiograph, W. J. Morton or William Herbert Rollins may have instead been first. William Herbert Rollins invented the first dental x-ray unit in the year (10) _____, although his equipment was never manufactured.

8. **1896**
9. **C. Edmund Kells**

10. **1896**

The first dentist to use radiographs for endodontic procedures was (11) _____. In the early days of dental radiography it was difficult to achieve uniform, standard, reproducible exposures because of the variability of the gases contained within the tube. The standard practice, as advocated by Kells, was to place the operator's hand between the tube and the fluoroscope to set the exposure time each time the machine was used. Needless to say, this practice resulted in the development of malignant lesions; before his death, Kells lost three fingers, his hand, and eventually his arm, from radiation overexposure.

11. **C. Edmund Kells**

It is for this reason that the inventor of the modern tungsten high-vacuum tube with a stable, reproducible output deserves a place in history. An employee of the General Electric Company, (12) _____, made his discovery in the year (13) _____. Unlike many of the early pioneers, Coolidge lived to the ripe old age of (14) _____.

12. **William D. Coolidge**
13. **1913**
14. **101**

The harmful effects of the Roentgen ray, as it was then known, were reported as early as April 10, 1896, only six months after Roentgen's first announcement. John Daniel reported that he had made a 1-hour head plate exposure on a Dr. William L. Dudley. (15) _____ fell out from the spot where Dr. Dudley was exposed to the (16) _____. Of course, this was not immediately perceived as harmful; radiation continued to be used for the removal of unwanted hair for some (17) _____ years following that report.

In the early days of dental radiography, all intraoral films were hand-wrapped by the operator or his assistant. The (18) _____ Company is generally credited with manufacturing the first prewrapped intraoral films in the year (19) _____.

In that same year, the first American commercially manufactured dental x-ray machine was made by the (20) _____ _____ Company at a cost of about $300.00. Though Kells was certainly one of the best-known early pioneers of dental radiography, Dr. (21) _____ _____ of San Francisco, California, has been hailed as the father of modern dental radiography. Among his many achievements, he developed the (22) _____ _____ technique. In 1924, Dr. (23) ____ _____ of Indianapolis, Indiana, invented the bite-wing film and wrote the first (24) _____ _____. Although Coolidge invented his tube in 1913, it was not until 1923 that a miniature version of the tube was placed inside the head of an x-ray machine and immersed in oil. This was the precursor of all modern dental x-ray machines. It was manufactured by the (25) _____ _____, which eventually became the (26) _____. This machine was wall-mounted, had a fully adjustable arm, a remote timer switch, and an open-ended cone, and was capable of exposures as long as 10 seconds.

Some of the modern practitioners who deserve a place in history include Dr. Fred M. Medwedeff, who in 1960 developed the (27) _____ technique and Dr. William Updegrave, who developed the (28) _____ _____ technique for both regular and rectangular collimation. Dr. Updegrave also developed the temporomandibular joint (29) _____ _____. Both of these techniques have gained wide acceptance and are commonly used today.

15. hair
16. radiation

17. 40

18. Eastman Kodak

19. 1913

20. American X-Ray Equipment

21. F. Gordon Fitzgerald

22. long-cone paralleling

23. Howard Riley Raper

24. dental radiology textbook

25. Victor X-Ray Corporation of Chicago

26. General Electric X-Ray Corporation

27. rectangular collimation

28. extension long-cone paralleling

29. angle board

Though the first panoramic radiograph was published by Prof. (30) _____ of Helsinki, Finland, the first commercially produced panoramic x-ray machine was the (31) _____, manufactured by the (32) _____ _____ Company. Much of the early work leading to the development of this machine was done by John W. Kampula, George Dickson, and Dr. Donald Hudson. It is generally agreed that the father of panoramic radiography is (33) _____. Dr. (34) _____ of Japan was the first to use the term *orthopantomograph* to describe the panoramic film.

30. **Yrjo V. Paatero**

31. **Panorex**
32. **S. S. White**

33. **Prof. Paatero**
34. **Eiko Sairenji**

Sample Examination Questions

1. The first dentist to take intraoral radiographs on a living patient was:

   A. W. G. Morton.
   B. C. Edmund Kells.
   C. Roentgen.
   D. Coolidge.

1. B

2. Which of the following statements is true?

   A. In 1895, William Crookes of Germany designed the first vacuum tube.
   B. William Crookes of England was one of the main investigators who modified the original Geissler tube.
   C. Roentgen designed the first vacuum tube.
   D. Kells was the first to discover x rays.

2. B

3. _____ depends on the differential absorption of x rays traversing an object and emerging to expose an x-ray film and produce an image.

   A. Roentgenology.
   B. Radiology.
   C. Radiography.
   D. Radioactivity.

3. C

4. X rays were discovered in:

   A. 1870.
   B. 1875.
   C. 1895.
   D. 1905.

4. C

5. X rays were discovered by:

   A. Geissler.
   B. Crookes.
   C. Roentgen.
   D. Walkhoff.

5. C

6. The first x-ray films had to be handled with extreme care because they were:

   A. Too flexible.
   B. Made of an emulsion on a celluloid base.
   C. Made of an emulsion on a glass plate.
   D. Made of an emulsion on a sheet of rubber.

6. C

7. The dentist credited with developing the bite-wing technique is:

   A. Howard Raper.
   B. Otto Walkhoff.
   C. Myron Kasle.
   D. Irving Lehr.

7. A

8. The dentist credited with developing the long-cone paralleling technique is:

   A. Olaf E. Langland.
   B. Donald Hudson.
   C. Myron Kasle.
   D. F. Gordon Fitzgerald.

8. D

9. The father of panoramic radiography is:

   A. Donald Hudson.
   B. Fred Musaph.
   C. Yrjo V. Paatero.
   D. S. S. White.

9. C

10. The first dental radiology textbook was written by:

    A. Olaf Langland.
    B. Leroy Ennis.
    C. Howard Raper.
    D. Myron Kasle.

10. C

SECTION 16

FINAL EXAMINATION REVIEW

Review Questions: Part 1

INSTRUCTIONS: Select the most correct answer for each question.

1. The x-ray beam is directed toward the patient's face with the:

   A. Tube.
   B. Cone.
   C. Collimator.
   D. Transformer.

   1. B

2. X rays are produced in the _____ of the dental x-ray unit.

   A. Tube.
   B. Cone.
   C. Collimator.
   D. Transformer.

   2. A

3. The x-ray beam collimator is usually constructed of:

   A. Copper.
   B. Aluminum.
   C. Lead.
   D. Plastic.

   3. C

4. X-ray beam filters used in dental radiology are most often made of:

   A. Plastic.
   B. Aluminum.
   C. Copper.
   D. Lead.

   4. B

5. The lead foil found in a typical Type-2 film packet:

   A. Absorbs some radiation passing through the film packet.
   B. Confuses the operator.
   C. Softens the emulsion.
   D. Acts as an intensifying screen.
   E. Reduces the developing time for the latent image.

   5. A

6. Radiographic films become stained because they are: 6. D

    (1) Developed in oxidized developer.
    (2) Stored at a high temperature.
    (3) Inadequately rinsed in water.
    (4) Stored in a lead container.
    (5) Excessively fixed.
A. 2 and 4.
B. 4 and 5.
C. 1, 2, and 3.
D. 1, 3, and 5.
E. All of the above.

7. The smaller the focal or target area, the better the radiographic: 7. D

A. Intensity.
B. Density.
C. Radiolucency.
D. Detail.

8. X rays were discovered: 8. B

    (1) After the first world war.
    (2) Before Lindbergh's flight (1927).
    (3) After the Bank Panic of 1890.
    (4) Prior to the assassination of President Lincoln.
A. 1 and 2.
B. 2 and 3.
C. 2 and 4.
D. 3 and 4.

9. Which of the following will minimize secondary or scatter radiation? 9. D

    (1) Lead backing in film packets.
    (2) Cassette grids.
    (3) Collimation.
    (4) Added filters.
A. 1 and 2.
B. 1 and 3.
C. 3 and 4.
D. All of the above.

10. Limiting the size of the x-ray beam is achieved by using a: 10. C

A. Pointed plastic cone.
B. Open-ended clear plastic cone.
C. Lead collimator.
D. Aluminum collimator.
E. None of the above.

11. The least diagnostically helpful waves of x-ray energy that are removed during filtration are characterized as:

   A. Short waves.
   B. Long waves.
   C. Beta waves.
   D. Proton waves.

11. **B**

12. Adumbration is another name for:

   A. Crooked roots.
   B. A television police show.
   C. Fused teeth.
   D. Cervical burnout.
   E. A genetic manifestation of teeth found in the Adams family.

12. **D**

13. Primary radiation comes from the x-ray:

   A. Cone.
   B. Transformer.
   C. Autotransformer.
   D. Tube.

13. **D**

14. Electromagnetic radiation includes such things as:

   (1) Protons.
   (2) Radio waves.
   (3) Gamma rays.
   (4) Visible light.
   (5) Electrons.
   A. 1, 2, and 4.
   B. 2, 3, and 4.
   C. 2, 3, and 5.
   D. 3, 4, and 5.
   E. 1, 3, 4, and 5.

14. **B**

15. The panoramic radiograph is:

   (1) Used as a screening film.
   (2) A film that surveys the maxilla and mandible.
   (3) A very fine image-detail film.
   (4) Used to improve image definition.
   A. 1 and 2.
   B. 1, 2, and 4.
   C. 1, 3, and 4.
   D. 2, 3, and 4.
   E. All of the above.

15. **A**

16. Which of the following describe x rays?

    (1) They are particulate in nature.
    (2) They are homogenous (have the same wavelengths).
    (3) They are able to curve around corners.
    (4) They are able to affect photographic film.
    (5) They are able to change biologic systems.

  A. 1 and 3.
  B. 3 and 5.
  C. 4 and 5.
  D. 1, 2, and 4.
  E. 2, 4, and 5.

16. C

17. Another name for the small spot on the face of the anode is the:

  A. Cup.
  B. Filament.
  C. Core.
  D. Base.
  E. Target.

17. E

18. Limiting the size of the x-ray beam to that required to expose the film is achieved by:

  A. Collimation.
  B. Filtration.
  C. Absorption.
  D. Changing the size of the film.

18. A

19. The longer the x-ray wavelength:

  A. The more penetrating the x-ray photons.
  B. The less penetrating the x-ray photons.
  C. The less absorbing the x-ray photons.
  D. The wavelength does not affect penetration.

19. B

20. When the milliamperage of the x-ray unit is increased from 10 to 15 mA, to maintain the same radiographic density it is necessary to:

  A. Increase the exposure time.
  B. Decrease the exposure time.
  C. Decrease the developing time.
  D. Do nothing; film density will remain the same.

20. B

21. One geometric factor or principle of shadow casting that will decrease the penumbra (increase sharpness) of the radiographic image is a:

    A. Short source-object distance.
    B. Long object-film distance.
    C. Long source-object distance.
    D. Large focal spot.

21. **C**

22. One geometric factor or principle of shadow casting that will increase the penumbra (reduce sharpness) of the radiographic image is a:

    A. Short object-film distance.
    B. Short source-object distance.
    C. Long source-object distance.
    D. Small focal spot.

22. **B**

23. The short open-ended, shielded-cone exposure time is .2 second, and the long open-ended, shielded-cone exposure time is .7 second (all other exposure and film factors remain constant). The patient will receive:

    A. Less radiation with the short cone.
    B. Essentially the same amount of radiation with either cone.
    C. More radiation with the long cone.
    D. More radiation with the short cone.

23. **B**

24. Which of the following demonstrates the indirect effect of x rays on a biologic system?

    A. Chromosomal mutation.
    B. Chromosomal break.
    C. Enzyme inactivation.
    D. Hydrogen peroxide production.

24. **D**

25. When an exposed radiograph is placed in the developing solution:

    A. The time it remains in solution is determined by the temperature of the solution.
    B. The unexposed silver bromide is removed.
    C. The image of the film becomes stabilized.
    D. The time it remains in solution is determined by the time it takes for the image to appear.

25. **A**

26. The x-ray operator is permitted to hold the film during exposure if:

   A. The patient is handicapped.
   B. The patient is mentally ill.
   C. The patient is a child.
   D. The operator is never permitted to hold the film during exposure.

26. D

27. Which of the following radiographic film codes would you use for an adult interproximal radiograph similar to those taken in a clinic?

   A. 1.1.
   B. 1.2.
   C. 2.0.
   D. 2.2.
   E. 3.4.

27. D

28. Dental radiographic film has a special code number to indicate the film function (purpose) and the size (dimensions) of the film. A box of film with a code designation of *3.4* would indicate films of an appropriate size for:

   A. Periapical radiographs.
   B. Occlusal radiographs.
   C. Interproximal radiographs.
   D. Pedodontic periapical radiographs.

28. B

29. The source of electrons used to produce x rays within the x-ray tube is controlled by the:

   A. Temperature of the filament (cathode).
   B. Temperature of the target (anode).
   C. X-ray time.
   D. Kilovoltage-adjustment knob.

29. A

30. Which of the following is the best method of reducing your exposure as an x-ray operator?

   A. Stand at least 6 feet away from the tube head when making an exposure.
   B. Stand behind an appropriate barrier or outside the room.
   C. Never hold films in the patient's mouth.
   D. Never hold or stabilize the tube head during exposures.
   E. All of the above.

30. E

31. Which of the following is known as the unit of dose equivalent?

A. Roentgen (R).
B. rad (radiation absorbed dose).
C. rem (roentgen equivalent mammal).
D. RBE (radiobiologic equivalent).
E. Gray (Gy).

31. C

32. Which of the following units of radiation measurement is defined as 100 ergs/gm of tissue?

A. Roentgen (R).
B. rad.
C. rem (roentgen equivalent mammal).
D. RBE (radiobiologic equivalent).
E. Gray (Gy).

32. B

33. The pointed plastic cone is not recommended for intra-oral radiography because it:

(1) Only comes in one length (short) and therefore cannot be used with the paralleling principle.
(2) Increases somatic exposure to the face and eyes.
(3) Increases scattered radiation to the reproductive organs.
(4) Is difficult to align accurately with the film.
(5) Is difficult to visualize the central ray.

A. 2 and 3.
B. 1, 2, and 4.
C. 1, 3, and 4.
D. 1, 2, 3, and 5.
E. All of the above.

33. A

34. The lead apron is primarily useful in reducing:

A. Reproductive-organ exposure due to scattered radiation.
B. Reproductive-organ exposure from the primary beam.
C. Somatic-tissue exposure to the face and neck.
D. All of the above.

34. A

35. The maximum permissible dose (MPD) can best be defined as:

    A. The amount of radiation just below the genetic mutation threshold.
    B. The amount of radiation that will produce minor genetic effects, but no somatic tissue effects.
    C. The amount of radiation that will not produce any serious deleterious effects.
    D. The amount of radiation that will produce both genetic and somatic effects.
    E. The amount of radiation a person may receive without lethal consequences.

35. C

36. Proper time-temperature processing of radiographs is essential to minimize patient exposure because it:

    A. Prevents overdeveloping radiographs that are routinely overexposed.
    B. Assures a diagnostic image with minimum amounts of radiation.
    C. Routinely develops film to a specific predetermined diagnostic density regardless of exposure or kilovoltage.
    D. Minimizes film fog from scattered radiation.

36. B

37. Which of the following factors will reduce the patient's somatic exposure by the greatest amount?

    A. Lead apron.
    B. Short pointed plastic cone.
    C. Short open-ended cone.
    D. Long open-ended cone with lead liner.
    E. Long lead-lined rectangular cone.

37. E

38. Which of the following statements correctly describes the latent period for radiation-induced bioeffects?

    (1) The time lapse between irradiation and the manifestation of specific biologic signs of tissue damage.
    (2) The time lapse between doses of irradiation to patients undergoing radiation therapy.
    (3) The time lapse from the time the exposure switch is depressed until the x rays are produced.
    (4) The length of the latent period depends on the amount and type of radiation given.
    (5) The length of the latent period is always constant, regardless of tissue or radiation type.

A. 1.
B. 1 and 4.
C. 1 and 5.
D. 2, 3, and 4.
E. 2, 4, and 5.

39. The National Council on Radiation Protection has established maximum permissible dose (MPD) guidelines for occupationally exposed and nonoccupationally exposed individuals. The MPD for a nonoccupationally exposed individual is:

A. 0.2 rem/year.
B. 0.5 rem/year.
C. 1 rem/year.
D. 3 rem/year.
E. 5 rem/year.

40. The occupational MPD for a pregnant woman is:

A. 0 rem/year.
B. 0.5 rem/year.
C. 1 rem/year.
D. 5 rem/year.
E. 10 rem/year.

41. The amount of tissue damage following irradiation depends on:

A. The dose rate and intensity.
B. The area or volume of tissue irradiated.
C. The intensity of the exposure (chronic or acute).
D. The radiosensitivity of the tissue.
E. All of the above.

42. Which of the following will NOT reduce the somatic (facial) exposure of a patient during dental radiography?

    A. A short open-ended, lead-lined cone instead of a pointed plastic one.
    B. A long open-ended, lead-lined cone.
    C. Rectangular collimator.
    D. Speed D film.
    E. A lead apron.

42. E

43. The peak kilovoltage (kVp) in a dental x-ray unit is altered by adjusting the:

    A. High-voltage (step-up) transformer.
    B. Autotransformer.
    C. Milliamperage.
    D. Low-voltage (step-down) transformer.
    E. Exposure time.

43. B

44. Which of the following is a major factor in reducing operator exposure during dental radiographic procedures?

    A. Use high-kilovoltage techniques, because a shorter exposure time is required.
    B. Use low-kilovoltage techniques, because photons produced with these techniques are not as penetrating as high-kilovoltage photons.
    C. Do not use a pointed plastic cone.
    D. Stand at least 6 feet away from the tube head and avoid the primary beam.
    E. Have the patient wear a lead apron.

44. D

45. Which of the following does NOT describe the latent radiographic image?

    A. It is a minute speck of metallic silver.
    B. It is produced by the interaction of x-ray photons with silver halide salts.
    C. It may be called the invisible radiographic image.
    D. It is made visible only after processing.
    E. It may be visible prior to developing and processing.

45. E

46. The two major purposes of the developing solution are to:

    A. Shrink emulsion and promote removal of unexposed crystals.
    B. Soften emulsion and develop silver halide crystals without a latent image.
    C. Soften emulsion and develop silver halide crystals containing a latent image.
    D. Prevent film fog and deterioration of developing agents.
    E. Remove developed silver halide crystals from the emulsion and harden the emulsion.

46. C

47. Of the following tissues, which is the most radiosensitive?

    A. Hematopoietic bone marrow.
    B. Skin.
    C. Muscle.
    D. Old bone.
    E. Nerve.

47. A

48. When reproductive organs are irradiated, the number of mutations will increase:

    A. Only if the dose exceeds the threshold value for that tissue.
    B. Following irradiation but the organs will return to their normal, nonmutated form within three weeks.
    C. In direct proportion to the amount of radiation.
    D. Inversely as the radiation dose rate and intensity decreases.

48. C

49. The target-film distance is:

    (1) One of the factors that determines the exposure time.
    (2) The only factor that determines the exposure time.
    (3) Increased to use lower kilovoltages.
    (4) Increased to make the beam size small enough to cover the film with less exposure to the patient.
    A. 1.
    B. 2.
    C. 4.
    D. 1 and 2.
    E. 2 and 4.

49. A

50. A very light radiograph may be caused by:

    (1) Too short an exposure time.
    (2) The leaded side of the film being toward the tube.
    (3) Developing solution that is too warm.
    (4) Removing the film from the fixing bath too soon.
    (5) The leakage of white light in the darkroom.

A. 1 and 2.
B. 1 and 3.
C. 1 and 4.
D. 2 and 3.
E. 2 and 5.
F. 3 and 4.
G. 3 and 5.
H. 4 and 5.

50. A

51. Excessively dark roentgenograms may be caused by:

    (1) Underdevelopment.
    (2) Excessive kilovoltage.
    (3) Excessive milliampere seconds.
    (4) Placing the film in the mouth backwards.

A. 1 and 2.
B. 1 and 3.
C. 1 and 4.
D. 2 and 3.
E. 2 and 4.
F. 3 and 4.

51. D

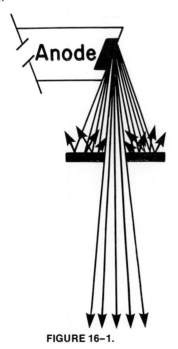

FIGURE 16–1.

52. Figure 16–1 illustrates the emanating radiation being restricted to a useful beam size. This is known as:

    A. Attenuation.
    B. Focusing.
    C. Collimation.
    D. Filtration.

52. C

53. The time lapse between irradiation and the biologic manifestation of radiation damage is called the:

    A. Lag-time interval.
    B. Latent period.
    C. Prodromal interval.
    D. Biologic manifestation interval.
    E. None of the above; radiation effects are immediate and there is no time lapse.

53. B

54. Dental developer solutions contain which of the following chemicals?

    (1) Sodium carbonate.
    (2) Barium sulfate.
    (3) Silver bromide.
    (4) Chrome alum.
    (5) Hydroquinone.
    A. 1 and 5.
    B. 2 and 4.
    C. 3 and 4.
    D. 1, 2, 4, and 5.
    E. All of the above.

54. A

55. Dental fixer solutions contain chemicals such as:

    (1) Sodium sulfate.
    (2) Acetic acid.
    (3) Chrome alum.
    (4) Hyposulfite (sodium thiosulfate).
    (5) Metol.
    A. 2, 3, and 4.
    B. 1, 2, 3, and 5.
    C. 1, 2, 4, and 5.
    D. 2, 3, 4, and 5.
    E. All of the above.

55. A

56. The best method for determining the sensitivity of dental x-ray film to x-radiation is to observe the:

   A. American National Standards Institute (ANSI) Speed Group A, B, C, D, E rating.
   B. ANSI Type 1.1, 1.2, or 3.4 codes.
   C. Manufacturer's brand name.
   D. Manufacturer's film code (e.g., DF-57, DF-58).
   E. None of the above; film sensitivity must be determined for each box in the office.

56. A

57. When x-radiation is absorbed by a biologic system, radiation damage is believed to be produced primarily by:

   (1) Ionization-induced inactivation of biologically active molecules (direct effects).
   (2) The production of heat.
   (3) Ionization of nonbiologically active molecules (water) to form toxic products that inactivate or damage biologically active molecules (indirect effects).

   A. 1 and 2.
   B. 1 and 3.
   C. 2 and 3.
   D. All of the above.

57. B

58. When x-ray photons are absorbed by silver halide crystals in the film emulsion:

   A. Nothing happens to the crystal until processing.
   B. A large grain of metallic silver is formed.
   C. A minute speck of metallic silver is formed.
   D. A deposit of solid bromide initiates image formation.

58. C

59. X rays are absorbed (lose their energy) by collision of the:

   A. Photon with the nucleus of the absorbing atom.
   B. Photon with the orbital electrons of the absorbing atom.
   C. High-speed electron with the nucleus.
   D. Photon with high-speed electrons.

59. B

60. The primary purpose of the lead diaphragm within the cone of the x-ray tube head is to:

A. Restrict the size and shape of the radiation beam.
B. Eliminate long-wavelength x-ray photons.
C. Prevent scattered radiation from the pointed cone tip.
D. Increase the penetrating qualities of the beam.
E. Reduce or eliminate tube head leakage.

60. A

61. The milliamperage adjustment control on the dental unit regulates the:

A. Temperature of the filament (cathode).
B. Penetration of the x-ray photon.
C. Quality of the x-ray beam produced.
D. Temperature of the anode.

61. A

62. The effective energy of the dental x-ray beam may be increased by:

A. Increasing the milliamperage.
B. Increasing the exposure time.
C. Increasing the kilovoltage.
D. Increasing the size (diameter) of the beam.
E. Decreasing the kilovoltage.

62. C

63. The aluminum filter in the x-ray tube head is used to:

(1) Preferentially absorb short-wavelength photons.
(2) Preferentially absorb long-wavelength photons.
(3) Increase the penetrating qualities of the beam.
(4) Decrease the penetrating qualities of the beam.
(5) Reduce the patient skin exposure.

A. 2 and 5.
B. 1, 3, and 5.
C. 1, 4, and 5.
D. 2, 3, and 5.
E. 2, 4, and 5.

63. D

64. Which of the following x-ray exposure factors will NOT increase the density of a dental radiograph? (Assume that the normal exposure factors for this unit are 80 kVp, 38/60 second, 10mA, and a 16-inch cone.)

A. kVp adjusted to 90 kVp.
B. kVp adjusted to 70 kVp.
C. Milliamperage set at 15 mA.
D. Exposure time adjusted to 42/60 second.
E. Cone length reduced from 16 to 8 inches.

64. B

65. At the atomic level, x-ray photons from the dental x-ray machine usually lose their energy through:

   A. Collisions with the absorbing atom's nucleus.
   B. Collisions with other photons.
   C. The Compton effect.
   D. The photoelectric effect.
   E. The bremsstrahlung effect.

65. D

66. When x rays are produced, approximately what per cent of the energy deposited in the target is actually converted into x-ray energy?

   A. 1% or less.
   B. 2%.
   C. 5%.
   D. 10%.
   E. 99%.

66. A

67. From a radiation protection standpoint, a patient will receive less somatic (facial) exposure from dental radiographs when which of the following is used?

   A. A short open-ended cone.
   B. A long open-ended (lead-lined) cone.
   C. A pointed plastic cone.
   D. A short open-ended (lead-lined) cone.
   E. A long rectangular (lead-lined) cone.

67. E

68. The National Council on Radiation Protection recommends that the useful diameter of the beam of radiation measured at the patient's skin should be no greater than:

   A. 1.75 inches.
   B. 2 inches.
   C. 2.5 inches.
   D. 2.75 inches.
   E. 3 inches.

68. E

69. According to the recommendations of the American Dental Association and the NCRP, a modern dental x-ray unit capable of producing more than 70 kVp must have a total aluminum filtration of at least:

   A. 0.5 mm aluminum.
   B. 1.0 mm aluminum.
   C. 1.5 mm aluminum.
   D. 2.0 mm aluminum.
   E. 2.5 mm aluminum.

69. E

70. The beam of radiation emitted from the x-ray tube head consists of:

    A. X-ray photons of many different energies and wavelengths.
    B. X-ray photons of uniform energies and wavelengths.
    C. X-ray photons of the same energy but different wavelengths.
    D. Cathode rays of varying intensities.
    E. A larger percentage of characteristic radiation than any other type of radiation.

70. A

71. When x rays are generated by the dental unit, the x-ray photons have:

    A. The same energy and wavelength.
    B. Many different energies and wavelengths.
    C. Only a few energies capable of penetrating dense tissues.
    D. Many different speeds.

71. B

72. X rays are primarily produced by the:

    A. Collision of high-speed electrons with the cathode.
    B. Deceleration of high-speed electrons by their interaction with the nuclei of the target atoms.
    C. Collision and interaction of photons with the nuclei of the target atoms.
    D. Collision of high-speed electrons with outer-orbital electrons of the target atoms.
    E. Collision of high-speed electrons with the nuclei of the target atoms.

72. B

73. X rays may best be described as:

    A. Minute bundles or packets of energy without rest mass.
    B. Small wavelike particles that have a finite rest mass.
    C. Small pieces of matter travelling in a straight line that have a finite rest mass.
    D. The same as electrons, only bigger.

73. A

74. What is the criterion for anatomic accuracy in a dental radiograph?

    A. The image of the tips of the molar cusps will be recorded with little or no occlusal surface showing.

    B. Open interproximal spaces; proximal contacts do not overlap unless the teeth are actually malposed.

    C. Distinct enamel caps and pulp chambers can be seen.

    D. In the maxillary molar region, the zygoma is not superimposed over the root apices of the maxillary molars.

    E. All of the above.

74. E

75. What causes reticulation?

    A. Dirty or contaminated wash water.

    B. Developer that is too strong.

    C. High humidity in the film storage area.

    D. Failure to agitate the film during development.

    E. Sudden extreme temperature changes in processing.

75. E

76. The use of a long cone as compared with a short cone:

    A. Minimizes enlargement of the image.

    B. Avoids overlapping.

    C. Prevents shape distortion.

    D. Causes blurring of the outline of the image.

    E. None of the above.

76. A

77. You want to change from a long-scale contrast film technique to a short-scale contrast film technique, maintaining the same density. What would you do?

    A. Increase the kVp and the mAs.

    B. Decrease the kVp and the mAs.

    C. Decrease the kVp and increase the mAs.

    D. Increase the kVp and decrease the mAs.

77. C

78. What is the greatest disadvantage of the bisecting-angle radiographic technique?

    A. Image distortion caused by film bending.

    B. Lack of definition of the image.

    C. Superimposition of zygoma over the apices of the maxillary posterior teeth.

    D. Shape distortion of the anatomic structure images.

    E. Magnification of the tooth images.

78. D

79. Why is the extension or so-called long cone a necessary adjunct to the paralleling or right-angle radiographic technique?

    A. To avoid magnification of the image.
    B. To avoid shape distortion of the image.
    C. To reduce secondary radiation.
    D. To facilitate correct vertical angulation of the cone.
    E. To avoid superimposition of anatomic structures.

79. A

80. When using the bisecting-angle radiographic technique, directing the x-ray beam perpendicular to the long axis of the teeth causes:

    A. Overlapping of tooth images.
    B. Foreshortening of tooth images.
    C. Magnification of tooth images.
    D. Elongation of tooth images.
    E. None of the above.

80. D

81. Which of the following could explain why your films are coming out too dark?

    (1) Unsafe safelight.
    (2) Light leaks in the darkroom.
    (3) Overfixation.
    (4) Overexposure.
    (5) Overdevelopment.
    (6) Underdevelopment.
    A. 2, 3, and 6.
    B. 1, 2, 3, and 4.
    C. 1, 2, 3, and 6.
    D. 1, 2, 4, and 5.
    E. All of the above.

81. D

82. The single most effective method of reducing patient somatic exposure is:

    A. The use of open-ended shielded cones.
    B. The use of a lead apron.
    C. The use of added filtration.
    D. Proper collimation.
    E. Speed D film.

82. E

83. Most genetic radiation exposure to human beings from man-made sources is the result of:

A. Emissions from nuclear reactors.
B. Nuclear testing.
C. Dental radiography.
D. Medical radiography.
E. Incorrectly adjusted color television sets.
F. Microwave ovens.

83. D

84. According to the American National Standards Institute (ANSI), dental films may be classified according to:

(1) Film speed and emulsion sensitivity.
(2) Film speed and inherent contrast.
(3) Film size (i.e., physical dimensions).
(4) Film size (i.e., silver halide grain size).
(5) Film function (i.e., use).
(6) Film function (i.e., inherent latent image–forming ability).

A. 2.
B. 1 and 3.
C. 1, 3, and 5.
D. 2, 4, and 5.
E. 2, 4, and 6.

84. C

85. A xeroradiographic plate uses _____ to produce images of objects.

A. Chemical solutions.
B. Electrostatic charges.
C. Alternating electrical current.
D. Magnetic charges.

85. B

86. In xeroradiography, which of the following is analogous to a film in conventional radiography?

A. Photoreceptor plate.
B. Special paper.
C. Copper plate.
D. Chemosensitive plate.

86. A

87. Which of the following statements is most correct in describing xeroradiography?

    (1) It is an extension of the autoradiographic technique using a scanner.

    (2) It produces a record of the structure of an object made on film by the object's own radioactivity.

    (3) It is a method of recording a photograph of the microscopic details in a thin specimen by means of soft x rays.

    (4) It is a method that produces a print of the densities produced by x rays on a specially prepared selenium plate which has been exposed to x rays.

    (5) It is a technique of activating the copying process with x rays, rather than ordinary light as done in a commercial copy machine.

  A. 1.
  B. 1 and 5.
  C. 2 and 3.
  D. 3 and 4.
  E. 4 and 5.

87. E

88. In panoramic radiography, the focal trough is the:

  A. Slit where excess radiation is filtered.
  B. Area that is in focus when the mA and kVp are adjusted.
  C. Zone of sharpness.
  D. Area that is collimated.

88. C

89. Which of the following most closely describes the strengths and weaknesses of panoramic radiographs versus intraoral dental radiographs?*

  A. Panoramic radiographs show the entire facial complex on one film, but the image outline on the entire radiograph is distinct and sharp on all patients.
  B. Panoramic radiographs use intensifying screens and screen-type film, and the images are not magnified due to decreased object-film distance.
  C. Panoramic radiographs use nonscreen exposure film and usually produce overlapping of tooth contacts in the bicuspid and molar areas.
  D. Panoramic radiographs are made extraorally and are a good screening device but they do not show the detail of intraoral radiographs as far as caries activity, periodontal membrane changes, lamina dura changes, and detail of trabeculation.

89. D

---

*From Council on Dental Materials and Devices. *JADA* 94:147, 1977.

Review Questions: Part 2

INSTRUCTIONS: Place a "T" for each true statement or an "F" for each false statement in the space provided.

1. The latent image is seen on the x-ray film after developing but before fixing. _____

    1. **F**

2. The rad is the amount of x-radiation that will produce (in 1 cc of air at standard temperature and pressure) ions carrying a charge of one electrostatic unit of either sign (positive or negative). _____

    2. **F**

3. In oral diagnostic radiography, the half-value layer of the beam is generally 5 mm of aluminum. _____

    3. **F**

4. A heterogeneous beam and a monochromatic beam have similar radiographic properties if they have the same half-value layer. _____

    4. **T**

5. Apart from the properties of the target material, the use of the line-focus principle allows for an increased number of x-ray photons to be produced with less heat per unit area. _____

    5. **T**

6. Photons of x-radiation are corpuscular in nature and have a wavelength of 10 to 15 angstroms. _____

    6. **F**

7. A longer latent period is usual with severe radiation doses. _____

    7. **F**

8. The minimum distance between the operator and the source of radiation should be six yards. _____

    8. **F**

9. When the lingual cusp tips are superimposed on the buccal cusp tips, the lingual cusp tips usually appear more opaque. _____

9. T

10. If a radiographic film is completely exposed and processed, it will be pitch black. _____

10. T

11. Screen film is generally used to reduce exposure time; it is the most common type of extraoral film. _____

11. T

12. Screen film is more sensitive to fluorescent light than to x rays. _____

12. T

13. Radiation may affect a person's own somatic cells as well as his genetic cells. _____

13. T

14. Characteristic radiations are used to identify chemical elements. _____

14. T

15. Dimensional distortion is inherent in the bisecting-angle technique. It may, in a multirooted tooth, produce elongation of some roots and foreshortening of others within the same radiographic image. _____

15. T

16. At present, the average individual exposure to radiation, including medical radiation, should not exceed 10 roentgens by age 30. _____

16. T

17. In all dental public health surveys, x rays are recommended because of our medicolegal responsibility to examine all patients completely. _____

17. F

18. The basic effects of ionization are molecular alteration and the production of new chemicals, such as enzymes. _____

18. T

19. Cell death usually occurs at the interphase of the cell cycle. _____

20. The central ray consists of photons that travel at the very center of the radiation cone, emerging from the window of the x-ray tube. _____

21. Young bone is more sensitive to radiation than mature bone. _____

22. In dental x-ray machines, line focus is produced by placing the target at an angle of 27°. _____

23. The inherent filtration in an x-ray machine consists of aluminum disks that filter out long, nonpenetrating x-ray photons in the beam. _____

24. A collimated beam is produced mainly by the use of a long cone. _____

25. Because of the inverse square law, the use of a long cone requires a greater exposure time if mA and kVp remain constant. Nevertheless, the use of the long cone is associated with less radiation exposure to the patient than the rectangular cone. _____

26. The thin sheet of lead foil in the film packet may, under certain circumstances, produce an image on the processed film. _____

27. In a monochromatic beam, all photons are of the same wavelength. _____

28. X rays interact with matter by both direct and indirect methods. _____

19. F

20. T

21. T

22. F

23. F

24. F

25. F

26. T

27. T

28. T

29. In general, the use of the long-cone paralleling technique with rectangular collimation will result in a reduction of absorbed radiation to the patient. _____

29. T

30. The development of eye cataracts as a consequence of exposure to ionizing radiation apparently follows a non-linear, threshold type of response. _____

30. T

31. The tissues most susceptible to ionizing radiation are blood-forming tissues and reproductive cells. _____

31. T

32. Leukemia is one disease that is considered a possible consequence of overexposure to ionizing radiation, especially long-term, low-dose exposures. _____

32. T

33. Genetic mutations (from any cause) are generally considered to be repairable, given enough recovery time. _____

33. F

34. In general, the more highly differentiated (specialized) the tissue, the more sensitive it is to ionizing radiation. _____

34. F

35. The bone marrow dose of radiation in panoramic radiography is less than 5% of the mandibular bone marrow dose received in a conventional series of periapical radiographs. _____

35. T

36. Dental radiographs that subject the cornea to radiation will normally result in cataract formation. _____

36. F

37. Regardless of how small the amount of radiation used for dental diagnostic purposes, some degree of risk is involved. _____

37. T

38. The risk of developing leukemia from dental radiography is not any greater than the risk associated with exposure to natural environmental levels of background radiation. _____

39. A conventional series of periapical radiographs results in a smaller bone marrow absorbed dose than extraoral radiography. _____

40. The number of lateral cephalometric radiographs required to double the leukemia risk would be in excess of 300. _____

41. The number of panoramic radiographs required to double the leukemia risk would be in excess of 200. _____

42. If the doubling dose (the dose required to double the risk) for bone marrow cancers is 0.8 rad, 51 conventional periapical radiographic surveys would be required to double the leukemia risk. _____

43. If the background radiation dose to the bone marrow is 87 mrem per year, then a conventional series of periapical radiographs is comparable to approximately nine weeks of background exposure. _____

44. The average background radiation dose to the bone marrow is 87 mrem per year. On this basis, the amount of bone marrow radiation received from panoramic radiography is comparable to one to two weeks of background radiation. _____

45. Lateral cephalometric radiography results in a bone marrow dose comparable to radiation doses received in panoramic radiography. _____

38. T

39. F

40. T

41. T

42. T

43. T

44. T

45. T

46. The signs and symptoms produced by a radiation dose of 700 R to a finger and 700 R to the whole body would be the same. _____   **46. F**

47. X rays were discovered by William Coolidge. _____   **47. F**

48. mA and exposure time are factors that directly relate to the number of electrons that will strike the target in a given exposure. _____   **48. T**

49. The number of electrons available for the production of x rays is controlled by the temperature of the filament. _____   **49. T**

50. The use of the line-focus principle causes a decrease in the size of the effective focal spot. _____   **50. T**

51. The focusing cup at the anode directs the electrons to hit the target. _____   **51. F**

52. The speed of the electrons as they travel from the filament to the target is unimpeded by the gases present in the tube. _____   **52. F**

53. The cathode-anode circuit is a high-voltage circuit and is controlled mainly by the mA setting. _____   **53. F**

54. Glandular epithelium is more sensitive than all other types of epithelium. _____   **54. F**

55. The latent period is the amount of time between the exposure of the organism to radiation and the time of recovery. _____   **55. F**

56. X rays, gamma rays, alpha particles, and beta particles are all forms of radiation belonging to the same family of electromagnetic radiation. _____

56. F

57. X rays are absorbed by solid and liquid matter but not by gases. _____

57. F

58. The shorter the wavelength of x-radiation, the more energetic the x-ray photon and the greater its penetration power. _____

58. T

59. The dental x-ray machine is a highly efficient system, with more than 99% of the electrical energy converted to x-radiation. _____

59. F

60. The fundamental process of x-ray production is the abrupt stopping of high-speed electrons. _____

60. T

61. X rays are produced in an x-ray machine primarily by the conversion of electromagnetic energy to the kinetic energy of mass in motion. _____

61. F

62. As object thickness increases, it is often advisable to use lower kVp to obtain greater penetration. _____

62. F

63. The accuracy of the impulse timers found on new x-ray machines is not better than 1/10 second. _____

63. F

64. A closed-ended cone is no longer used as a positioning indicator because secondary radiation may be produced by the interaction of x-ray photons and the cone material. _____

64. T

65. Scatter and secondary radiation remain within the operatory for at least 15 seconds after the primary beam has been turned off. _____

65. F

66. Scatter radiation must be regarded as whole-body radiation. _____

66. T

67. A Geiger counter can be used to detect alpha-, beta-, and and gamma-type radiations. _____

67. T

68. Roentgen is a term used to express tissue dosage resulting from exposure to x rays. _____

68. F

69. True distortion is the result of the relations among the central beam of the x ray, the object being radiographed, and the film. _____

69. T

70. Magnification or false distortion can be decreased by increasing the target-film distance and decreasing the object-film distance. _____

70. T

71. Generally, underexposed radiographs lack contrast; overexposed radiographs also lack contrast. _____

71. T

72. When a short cone is replaced by a long cone, the density decreases and the sharpness increases. _____

72. T

73. The patient receives decreased radiation when using the short-cone technique because of decreased exposure time. _____

73. F

74. The indirect effect of radiation is most often mediated through the water molecule. _____

74. T

75. High contrast occurs when there are few shades of gray in a radiograph. _____

75. T

76. Density is a measure of the degree of blackness in a radiograph. _____

76. T

77. A short cone produces a longer image of a tooth than a long cone. _____

77. T

78. Developer marks leave black areas on a film. _____

78. T

79. All other factors being equal, it will take less total x-ray exposure time of a screen-film combination to produce a film density of 1.8 than it will with nonscreen film. _____

79. T

80. Provided the safelight is properly installed, it is not necessary to match the brand of light to specific film brands. _____

80. F

81. When x rays hit the film emulsion, they convert the metallic silver particles in the emulsion to black silver bromide crystals. _____

81. F

82. The image seen in films used with intensifying screens is slightly less sharp than that seen in nonscreen films. _____

82. T

83. The major ingredient of the fixer is Metol. _____

83. F

Review Questions: Part 3

INSTRUCTIONS: Match the statement in Column A with the *most appropriate* statement in Column B. Do not use any statement in Column B more than once. There may be more statements in Column B than are needed to complete the matching.

1.

Column A		Column B			
___1.	tungsten filament	A.	window	1.	C
___2.	molybdenum cup	B.	anode	2.	E
___3.	tungsten button	C.	cathode	3.	B
___4.	copper rod	D.	thermal conductor	4.	D
___5.	lead washer	E.	focusing device	5.	G
___6.	aluminum disk	F.	filter	6.	F
		G.	collimator		

2.

Column A		Column B			
___1.	elon	A.	preservative	1.	E
___2.	hydroquinone	B.	oxidizer	2.	D
___3.	sodium sulfite	C.	removes silver bromide	3.	A
___4.	sodium carbonate			4.	H
___5.	potassium bromide	D.	builds up contrast slowly	5.	I
___6.	sodium thio-sulfate	E.	brings out image quickly	6.	C
___7.	potassium alum	F.	acidifier	7.	G
___8.	acetic acid	G.	shrinks and hardens gelatin	8.	F
		H.	activates developing solution		
		I.	prevents chemical fog		

	Column A		Column B		
3.	_____ 1.	herringbone pattern	A.	improper cone placement	1. **B**
	_____ 2.	partial image	B.	film placed backwards	2. **A**
	_____ 3.	overlapping			3. **D**
	_____ 4.	elongation	C.	vertical angle too acute	4. **C**
	_____ 5.	radiolucent spots	D.	horizontal angle off	5. **I**
	_____ 6.	radiopaque spots	E.	vertical angle too obtuse	6. **H**
	_____ 7.	black lightning streaks	F.	low humidity	7. **F**
	_____ 8.	crescent-shaped radiolucent mark	G.	depleted fixer	8. **O**
			H.	fixer artifact	
	_____ 9.	radiolucent fingerprint	I.	developer artifact	9. **L**
	_____10.	greenish yellow hue on film	J.	developer too hot	10. **G**
			K.	high temperature differential between solutions	
	_____11.	fogged film			11. **N**
	_____12.	film too dark	L.	fluoride contamination	12. **J**
	_____13.	film too light	M.	high humidity	13. **P**
	_____14.	orange-peel or shattered glass appearance of emulsion	N.	unsafe safelight	14. **K**
			O.	fingernail artifact	
			P.	developer exhausted	

	Column A		Column B			
4.	_____ 1.	development center	A.	acidic solution	1.	L
	_____ 2.	intraoral radiographic film	B.	silver bromide crystals	2.	E
	_____ 3.	latent image	C.	all silver is precipitated	3.	I
	_____ 4.	photosensitivity	D.	preservative contained in both developer and fixer	4.	B
	_____ 5.	produces swelling of emulsion			5.	O
	_____ 6.	fixer	E.	double emulsion	6.	A
	_____ 7.	radiopaque area on processed film	F.	hardener of the emulsion in the fixer solution	7.	K
	_____ 8.	potassium alum	G.	produced by inadequate angulation	8.	F
	_____ 9.	sodium sulfite			9.	D
	_____10.	radiolucent area on processed film	H.	restrainer in the developing solution	10.	C
			I.	may last for several years; is a collection of development centers		
	_____11.	elongation			11.	G
	_____12.	cervical burnout			12.	N
	_____13.	potassium bromide	J.	produced by low-kV machines	13.	H
	_____14.	short-scale contrast	K.	no silver is precipitated	14.	J
	_____15.	foreshortening			15.	M
	_____16.	long-scale contrast	L.	area where Ag$^+$ and Br$^-$ are affected by x rays	16.	P
			M.	produced by excessive vertical angulation		
			N.	may mimic caries		
			O.	sodium carbonate		
			P.	produced by high-kV machines		

	Column A		Column B			
5.	_____ 1.	100 ergs per gram	A.	vertical angulation	1.	**L**
	_____ 2.	tungsten filament	B.	ANSI Group D	2.	**J**
	_____ 3.	cracked emulsion	C.	rotating anode	3.	**H**
	_____ 4.	elongation	D.	roentgen	4.	**A**
	_____ 5.	decreased ex- posure time	E.	reduces facial exposure	5.	**B**
	_____ 6.	400 mAs	F.	better definition	6.	**C**
	_____ 7.	collimation	G.	strontium 90	7.	**E**
	_____ 8.	tungsten target	H.	crescent-shaped	8.	**I**
	_____ 9.	radioactive iodine		marks	9.	**M**
	_____10.	one electrostatic unit per cubic centimeter	I.	high atomic number	10.	**D**
			J.	thermionic emission effect		
			K.	erythema dose		
			L.	rad		
			M.	gamma rays		

INSTRUCTIONS: Read the directions for each question.

6. Contrast and density of radiographic films are important factors in diagnostic radiography. Select the factor for each statement that best applies (factors may be used more than once).

Statement	Factor	
_____ 1. defined as a logarithm	A. contrast	1. B
_____ 2. increased with decreased penumbra	B. density	2. D
_____ 3. influenced by change in kilovoltage	C. contrast and density	3. C
_____ 4. influenced by change in target-film distance	D. does not apply to contrast and density	4. B
_____ 5. enables image details to become visible because of tonal relationship		5. A
_____ 6. influenced by change in milliamperage seconds		6. B
_____ 7. scatter radiation causes decrease		7. A
_____ 8. may be long scale or short scale		8. A
_____ 9. refers to overall blackness of film		9. B
_____ 10. affected by temperature of developer		10. C
_____ 11. influenced by movement of source		11. D
_____ 12. influenced by the atomic numbers, densities, and thicknesses of tissues being radiated		12. C

7. Match the radiation type with the characteristics (radiation types may be used more than once).

Characteristics	Radiation Type		
_____ 1. possesses mass	A. x-radiation	1.	**B and C**
_____ 2. positively charged	B. alpha radiation	2.	**B**
_____ 3. negatively charged	C. beta radiation	3.	**C**
_____ 4. ionizing radiation		4.	**A, B, and C**
_____ 5. no electric charge		5.	**A**
_____ 6. most penetrating radiation of the three		6.	**A**
_____ 7. least penetrating radiation of the three		7.	**B**

8. The following numbered phrases all relate to radiation's biologic effects.
   1. threshold effect
   2. nonthreshold effect
   3. direct-effect theory
   4. indirect-effect theory
   5. whole-body irradiation
   6. local-area irradiation

For each of the following statements match the most appropriate numbered phrase.

A. Radiation damage is produced by photons striking and inactivating (damaging) biologically active molecules. _____   **A. 3**

B. Genetic or chromosomal mutations increase in direct proportion to the amount of radiation received. _____   **B. 2**

C. Dental effects of ionizing radiation are primarily a result of _____.   **C. 6**

D. The development of carcinogenesis or leukemia among occupationally exposed persons is primarily a result of low-dose _____.   **D. 5**

E. The production of H_2O_2 as a result of the ionization of water produces damage by the _____.   **E. 4**

F. The erythema dose is a _____.   **F. 1**

Review Questions: Part 4

INSTRUCTIONS: Read each question carefully and select or calculate the correct answer.

1. A dentist has been exposing posterior periapical radiographs at 70 kVp, 15 mA, and 0.8 second at a 16-inch target-film distance. What would be the new exposure time if the milliamperage was changed to 10 mA and other factors remained the same?

   1. **1.2 seconds**
   $15 \text{ mA} \times 0.8 \text{ sec.} = 12 \text{ mAs}$
   $\dfrac{12 \text{ mAs}}{10 \text{ mA}} = 1.2 \text{ seconds}$

2. A dentist has been exposing posterior periapical radiographs at 75 kVp, 10 mA, and 0.3 second at an 8-inch target-film distance. What would be the new exposure time if the milliamperage was increased to 15 mA and other factors remained unchanged?

   2. **0.2 second**
   $10 \text{ mA} \times 0.3 \text{ sec} = 3 \text{ mAs}$
   $\dfrac{3 \text{ mAs}}{15 \text{ mA}} = 0.2 \text{ second}$

3. A dentist has been exposing posterior periapical radiographs at 70 kVp, 15 mA, and 0.20 second at an 8-inch target-film distance. What would be the new exposure time if he used a 16-inch target-film distance and other factors remained unchanged?

   3. **0.8 second**
   $\dfrac{8^2}{16^2} = \dfrac{0.20}{X}$
   $64X = 256 \ (0.20)$
   $X = \textbf{0.8 second}$

4. At 90 kVp and 15 mA at a target-film distance of 8 inches, the exposure time for a film is .50 second. Under the same conditions, what is the exposure time at 16 inches?

   4. **2.0 seconds**
   $\dfrac{8^2}{16^2} = \dfrac{0.5}{X}$
   $64X = 256 \ (0.5)$
   $64X = 128$
   $X = \dfrac{128}{64}$
   $X = \textbf{2.0 seconds}$

5. If mA and kVp are kept constant and the exposure time is 1 second with the 16-inch cone, what must the exposure time be if an 8-inch cone is used?

   A. .25 second.
   B. .5 second.
   C. 4 seconds.
   D. None of the above.

   5. **A**

6. In a given set of circumstances the mA is 10 and the exposure time is 1/4 second for an ideal exposure at 65 kVp. If the kVp is kept constant and the mA is set at 15, what will the new exposure time be?

   A. 1/8 second.
   B. 1/6 second.
   C. 23/60 second.
   D. None of the above.

6. B

7. Present exposure factors are: 8-inch cone, 10 mA, 80 kVp, 8/60 second exposure time, 375 mR exposure at cone tip. What will be the new exposure time if a 16-inch cone is used?

7. 32/60 second
$$\frac{8}{60} \times 4 = \frac{32}{60} \text{ second}$$
(The inverse square law–when you double the cone length you must quadruple the exposure time if all other factors remain constant.)

8. With the new exposure time calculated for the 16-inch cone in Question 7, what would be the new exposure at the cone tip?

   A. 93 mR.
   B. 187 mR.
   C. 375 mR.
   D. 750 mR.
   E. 825 mR.

8. C

9. Using the inverse square law, calculate the exposure at 16 inches if the original exposure at 8 inches was 500 mR. If you wanted to maintain the density on your radiograph (assuming all other factors constant), how much would you increase or decrease your exposure time?

   A. 125 mR; increase exposure time by four.
   B. 250 mR; increase exposure time by two.
   C. 500 mR; no increase or decrease in exposure time.
   D. 1000 mR; decrease exposure time by two.

9. A

10. Patient A is radiographed using a short open-ended cone with an exposure time of .2 second. Patient B is radiographed with a long, shielded, open-ended cone with an exposure time of .8 second. All other exposure and film factors remain the same, and films are processed according to the time-temperature method. Mounted radiographs are of similar quality and density. It may be assumed that:

   A. Patient A receives less exposure than Patient B.
   B. Patients A and B receive the same amount of radiation.
   C. Patient B receives four times more radiation than Patient A.
   D. Patient B's radiographs are being overexposed and underdeveloped.
   E. Patient A's radiographs are being underexposed and overdeveloped.

   10. B

11. A student using 70 kVp, 10 mA, and an 8-inch focal-film distance with corresponding exposure places the open-ended x-ray cone 4 inches from the skin while making a molar exposure. The resulting film will be:

   A. Overexposed because of the thermionic emission effect.
   B. Overexposed because of the inverse square law.
   C. Underexposed because of the excessive collimation.
   D. Underexposed because of the inverse square law.

   11. D

12. When using the paralleling radiographic technique, what would be the per cent of magnification of an object situated 1 inch from the film when the source-film distance is 16 inches?

   12. 6.6%

   $$\%M = \left(\frac{SFD}{SFD - OFD}\right) - 1 \times 100\%$$

   $$= \left(\frac{16}{16 - 1}\right) - 1 \times 100\%$$

   $$= 1.066 - 1 \times 100\%$$
   $$= 6.6\%$$

13. What would be the per cent of magnification of an object situated 1/2 inch from the film when the source-film distance is 8 inches?

   13. 6.6%

   $$\%M = \left(\frac{SFD}{SFD - OFD}\right) - 1 \times 100\%$$

   $$= \left(\frac{8}{8 - .5}\right) - 1 \times 100\%$$

   $$= \left(\frac{8}{7.5}\right) - 1 \times 100\%$$

   $$= 1.066 - 1 \times 100\%$$

   $$= 6.6\%$$

14. What would be the per cent of magnification of a tooth when the object-film distance is 1 inch, the distance from the object to the tip of the cone is 1/2 inch, and a short 8-inch cone is used?

14. 11.7%

$$\%M = \left(\frac{SFD}{SFD - OFD}\right) - 1 \times 100\%$$

$$SFD = 8 + .5 + 1 = 9.5$$

$$\%M = 11.7\%$$

15. If the length of an x-ray image of a tooth is 25 mm as measured on a radiograph using a 16-inch cone, a 1-inch object-film distance, and a 0.5-inch distance from the tip of the cone to the tooth, what is the actual length of the tooth?

15. 23.5 mm

$$\frac{\textbf{Actual length}}{\textbf{x-ray length}} = \frac{\textbf{SOD}}{\textbf{SFD}}$$

$$SOD = 16 + 0.5 = 16.5$$

$$SFD = 16 + 0.5 + 1 = 17.5$$

$$\frac{X}{25} = \frac{16.5}{17.5}$$

$$17.5X = 412.5$$

$$X = 23.5$$

16. You have been using a periapical film of Speed Group D and decide to change to a film of Speed Group A. To have a film of the same density, you should:

A. Increase the exposure six times.
B. Decrease the exposure one-sixth times.
C. Increase the exposure eight times.
D. Decrease the exposure one-eighth times.

16. C

17. You have a 28-year-old assistant who has been working in dental operatories with ionizing radiation since age 18. She has been exposing radiographs for the last four years. What would be her maximum permissible occupational accumulated dose? *NOTE*: She should *never* approach this dose if good radiation practices are used.

17. 50 rem

$$MPD = 5 (N - 18) \text{ rem}$$

$$= 5 (28 - 18)$$

$$= 50 \text{ rem}$$

18. A 50-year-old dental assistant has received an accumulated dose of 140 rems. The assistant has received:

    A. More than the maximum permissible accumulated dose.

    B. Less than the maximum permissible accumulated dose.

    C. The maximum permissible accumulated dose.

    D. An extremely lethal dose.

18. B

$MPD = 5 (N - 18)$ rem

$= 5 (50 - 18)$

$= 160$ rem

19. A dentist has been exposing posterior periapical radiographs at 70 kVp, 15 mA, and 0.8 second at a 16-inch target-film distance. What would be the new exposure time if the kilovoltage was changed to 80 kVp and other factors remained the same (mAs multiplying factor = 0.62*)?

*From Fuchs, A. W.: *Radiographic Exposure and Processing.* 2nd Edition. Charles C Thomas, 1969, p. 70.

19. 0.496 second

15 mA $\times$ **0.8 second**

$= 12$ mAs

12 mAs $\times$ 0.62*

$= 7.44$ mAs

$\dfrac{7.44 \text{ mAs}}{15 \text{ mA}} = 0.496$ second

20. A dentist has been exposing posterior periapical radiographs at 70 kVp, 15 mA, and 0.20 second at an 8-inch target-film distance. What would be his new exposure time if he changed to 85 kVp, 10 mA, and a 16-inch target film distance (mAs multiplying factor = 0.52*)?

*From Fuchs, A. W.: *Radiographic Exposure and Processing.* 2nd Edition. Charles C Thomas, 1969, p. 70.

20. 0.624 second

$$\dfrac{8^2}{16^2} = \dfrac{0.20}{X}$$

$64X = 256 (0.20)$

$X = 0.8$ second

15 mA $\times$ **0.8 second**

$= 12$ mAs

12 mAs $\times$ 0.52*

$= 6.24$ mAs

$\dfrac{6.24 \text{ mAs}}{10 \text{ mA}} = 0.624$ second

Review Questions: Part 5

INSTRUCTIONS: Carefully read the directions for each question.

1. Given the following graph of the spectrum of a dental
   x-ray beam, draw and label lines to indicate the effect of:
       (1) Increasing the mA.
       (2) Increasing the kVp.
       (3) Increasing the filtration.

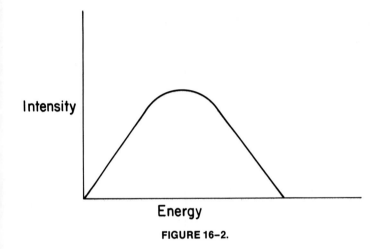

FIGURE 16–2.

1.

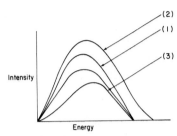

FIGURE 16–3. Answer.

2. Why is the temperature of the developing solution of
   critical importance if you are trying to maximize diagnostic information (refer to Figure 16–4)?

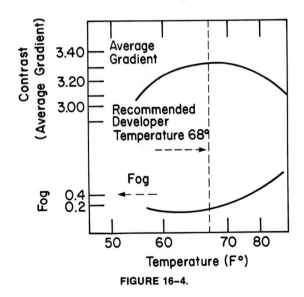

FIGURE 16–4.

2. **Most dental devel-
   oper solutions use
   hydroquinone,
   which works slowly
   in a maximum effici-
   ency range of 65 to
   70°F. Processing
   outside of this nar-
   row temperature
   range reduces the
   amount of black-
   ness of the proc-
   essed radiograph.**

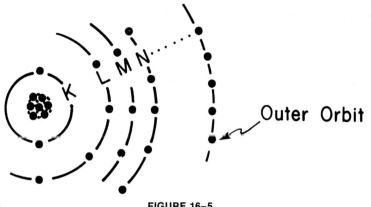

FIGURE 16–5.

3. Using Figure 16–5, answer the following questions.

   When we displace one electron from the outer orbit or shell, we have produced an (A) _____ .
   The larger fragment of this split has a net (B) _____ _____ charge and will tend to (C) _____ _____ .

4. If the x-ray machine operates at 50 kVp, we can displace K-orbit electrons:

   A. Only when we have a direct hit by a filament electron.
   B. With relatively great frequency and regularity.
   C. Never.
   D. And produce a burst of characteristic radiation.

Questions 5 through 9 refer to Figure 16–6, a diagram of an x-ray spectrum for a dental machine using a tungsten target. Briefly answer each question.

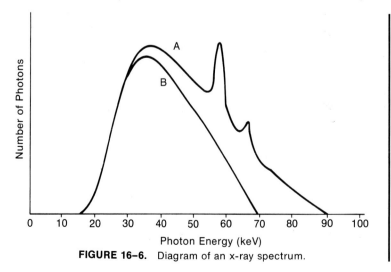

FIGURE 16–6. Diagram of an x-ray spectrum.

5. Which x-ray spectrum has the greatest penetrating power? _____

5. A

6. In Spectrum A, what do the spikes in the plot represent?
_____

6. characteristic x rays

7. X rays less than 20 keV in both plots are _____
_____

7. filtered out

8. The kilovoltage peak setting on the control panel of the machine producing Spectrum A is _____.

8. 90 kVp

9. Spectrum B does not show the spikes in the plot because
_____
_____.

9. the electron beam striking the anode does not have the kinetic energy to overcome the binding energy of the K shell of tungsten, which is 69.5 keV

10. Identify the appearance of a film after each of the following circumstances:

   A. Exposed to light, then processed. _____
   B. Processed without exposure to light or x ray. _____
   C. Exposed to an x-ray beam, then processed in fixer before developer. _____
   D. Stuck to another film during developing. _____
   E. Stuck to another film during fixing. _____
   F. Six months after inadequate washing following fixing. _____

10. A. black
    B. clear
    C. clear
    D. light area
    E. dark area
    F. brown

APPENDIX 1

REVIEW OF DEFINITIONS

1. _____: water in a transient, chemically reactive state created by absorbed ionizing radiations.

2. _____: an atomic particle, atom, or chemical radical bearing a positive or negative electrical charge; a molecular species that has lost or gained an electron; in solution, a hydrated ion results, so that ionization reactions followed by hydration can be very complex.

3. _____: two particles of opposite electrical charge; usually refers to the electron and the positive atomic residue that results from the interaction of an ionizing radiation photon with an orbital electron of an atom. The average energy required to produce an ion pair is approximately 33 eV (electron volt) in air.

4. _____: the process whereby a neutral atom or molecule acquires either a positive or negative charge.

5. _____: the radiation exposure required to produce in air 2.58×10^{-4} coulomb of ions of either charge per kilogram of air.

6. _____: a quantity of electrical charge that, if placed in a vacuum 1 centimeter from another unit charge of the same type and strength, will repel it with a force of 1 dyne.

7. _____: the amount of force that can accelerate a mass of 1 gram 1 centimeter per second.

8. _____: an energy absorption of 100 ergs per gram of any material.

9. _____: the work done by moving a body 1 centimeter against a force of 1 dyne.

10. _____: a unit of dose equivalent that represents a quantity of any radiation that produces the same biologic damage in man as the absorption of 1 roentgen of x-radiation or gamma radiation (X = dose (R) × QF).

11. _____: the inverse ratio of the absorbed dose from a test radiation type to that of a reference radiation required to produce the same stipulated effect.

1. activated water

2. ion

3. ion pair

4. ionization

5. roentgen

6. one electrostatic unit (esu)

7. dyne

8. rad

9. erg

10. rem

11. RBE (relative biologic effectiveness) (RBE for x rays, gamma rays, electrons, and beta particles = 1.0)

12. The following formula applies to dental radiography.

$$1 \text{ R} = \underline{\hspace{2cm}} = \underline{\hspace{2cm}}$$

13. \underline{\hspace{4cm}}: the kinetic energy gained by an electron falling through a potential difference of 1 volt.

14. \underline{\hspace{4cm}}: a random and permanent change in a gene.

15. \underline{\hspace{3cm}}: a series of narrow lead strips closely spaced on their edges and separated by spaces of low density material; used to prevent as much scattered radiation as possible from reaching the x-ray film during radiographic exposure.

16. \underline{\hspace{3cm}}: the material placed in the useful beam to preferentially absorb the less energetic (less penetrating) radiations.

17. \underline{\hspace{3cm}}: a redness of the skin or mucosa following exposure to certain irritants (heat, drugs, ultraviolet or ionizing radiation), due to congestion of the capillaries.

18. \underline{\hspace{3cm}}: a negatively charged elementary particle with a mass of 9.1×10^{-28} gram.

19. \underline{\hspace{3cm}}: any elementary particle with a rest mass intermediate in value between the masses of a proton and an electron.

20. \underline{\hspace{3cm}}: a fundamental particle with a mass equal to that of an electron and a positive charge equal to the negative charge of the electron.

21. \underline{\hspace{3cm}}: an elementary nuclear particle with a positive electrical charge and a rest mass equal to 1.007594 atomic mass units.

22. \underline{\hspace{3cm}}: an elementary particle having a rest mass of 1.00894 atomic mass units of no electrical charge; a component of the nucleus of all atoms except hydrogen.

23. \underline{\hspace{3cm}}: the energy possessed by a mass because of its motion.

24. \underline{\hspace{3cm}}: the rate (keV/micron) at which energy is released along the track of an ionizing particle traversing a medium.

12. 1 rad = 1 rem

13. electron volt (eV)

14. genetic mutation

15. grid

16. filter

17. erythema

18. electron

19. meson

20. positron

21. proton

22. neutron

23. kinetic energy

24. linear energy transfer (LET)

25. _____: radiation characteristic of particles with a low mass such as x rays, gamma rays, and electrons.

26. _____: a discrete unit of electromagnetic radiation or the amount of energy associated with a photon.

27. _____: a pattern of nonuniform density produced on screen films during radiographic exposure that is dependent on the screen type, and that results from the statistical fluctuation in the number of quanta per unit area absorbed by the intensifying screen.

28. _____: the energy of electromagnetic waves (radio waves, visible light, x rays, gamma rays, etc.).

29. _____: relative susceptibility of cells, tissues, organs, or organisms to the injurious action of radiation.

30. _____: energetic electrons resulting from Compton absorption of photons.

31. _____: radiation that, during passage through a substance, has been deviated in direction. It may also have been modified by an increase in wavelength. It is a form of secondary radiation.

32. _____: inelastic scattering of photons interacting with electrons in which incident photons are scattered with reduced energies; the remaining energy is given to the ejection of electrons (recoil electrons).

33. _____: a quantum of electromagnetic radiation.

34. _____: a spectral distribution of x rays ranging from low-energy photons to those produced by the peak kilovoltage applied across an x-ray tube; also means "braking radiation," referring to the sudden deceleration of electrons (cathode rays) as they strike the target in an x-ray tube.

25. low LET

26. quantum

27. quantum mottle

28. radiant energy

29. radiosensitivity

30. recoil electrons

31. scattered radiation

32. Compton (incoherent) scattering

33. photon

34. bremsstrahlung radiation

35. _____: forms of energy propagated by wave motion as photons or discrete quanta. The radiations have no matter associated with them. They differ widely in wavelength, frequency, and photon energy and have strikingly different properties. Covering an enormous range of wavelengths (10^{17} to 10^{-6} angstroms), they include radio waves, infrared waves, visible light, ultraviolet radiation, x rays, gamma rays, and cosmic radiation.

35. **electromagnetic radiation**

36. _____: particles or photons produced by the interaction of primary radiation with matter.

36. **secondary radiation**

37. _____: a secondary shadow that surrounds the periphery of the primary shadow. In radiography it is the blurred margin of an image detail.

37. **penumbra**

38. _____: excessive x-ray penetration of an object or part of an object producing a totally black, overexposed area on a radiograph.

38. **radiographic burn-out**

39. _____: a device used for converting an alternating current to a direct current; also used to prevent or limit the flow of current in the opposite direction.

39. **rectifier**

40. _____: an electrical device that alters the voltage of an alternating current by mutual induction between primary and secondary windings.

40. **transformer**

APPENDIX 2

ASPECTS OF THE
FUTURE OF RADIOLOGY

James W. Frazer

It is almost a truism that students are usually well prepared to use diagnostic equipment that is 10 years out of date; they will have to have considerable postgraduate learning to remain current in their field. Within the past 15 years, the various forms of panoramic radiography (also known as rotational radiography) have begun to enjoy acceptance as survey and facial structural analysis tools. The impact of tomographic imaging for cephalometry is increasingly being felt, but the process remains too expensive for all but large, central health institutions. Major developments in computer technology and image processing indicate that computed tomographic procedures can be made much less expensive than at present ($400,000 to $750,000), but it is dubious whether the CT scanner will ever be used in private offices in the near or distant future. Rotational radiology, on the other hand, could be used to produce three-dimensional or sliced formats of dental structures in the distant future and can be made available at an affordable price by private practitioners. With known advances in image enhancement technology, an attractive means of producing images of acceptable diagnostic quality with reduced radiation dose to the patient and practitioner is a possibility being actively pursued in several laboratories and manufacturing companies at the present time.

There are, however, energy forms other than x rays that can be utilized to form images of internal structures. At present, ultrasonic imaging and radiofrequency imaging are both being actively developed. Ultrasonic imaging is already being used in fetal diagnostic procedures, whereas radiofrequency imaging is still, at the moment, a laboratory curiosity. Both of these modalities require microprocessor-controlled image formation on a television screen or other electronic recording device. Ultrasound suffers from disadvantages because of the necessity of acoustically coupling the patient to the transducer, which may vary considerably, causing image distortion. On the other hand, several companies have developed acoustic phased arrays, which successfully scan internal organs in real time with real time image presentation so that functional organ descriptions can be made. Applications to oral radiologic procedures are beset with resolution limitations, but the problem seems tractable so that high resolution acoustic imaging of dental features in five to 10 years seems possible (sooner if Japanese electronics firms such as Toshiba continue at their present rate).

A leading resercher in radiofrequency imaging has already been successful in using nuclear magnetic resonance imaging to produce cross sections of the head, thoracic, and abdominal regions. The technique is uniquely applicable to tumor diagnosis since a chemical map is portrayed rather than the density map usually seen in present x rays. The chemical determinations, used for several years in organic chemistry as a means of chemical structure determination, are made possible by the fact that several naturally occurring nuclei (H^1, O^{17}, C^{13}, K^{40}, Ca^{45}) have odd nuclear spins, making them detectable by radiofrequency fields of an appropriate, known frequency when a known magnetic field is present. By application of a strong radiofrequency and observation of relaxation after its termination, unique information concerning biologic structure is determined. This measurement has been shown to have potential in tumor detection. Even crude laboratory scale systems now being used have resolutions on the order of 1 to 3 mm, and there is no real theoretical limit to this resolution. Development, however, will be expensive and time-consuming; commercial instruments will not be available for some years.

Another form of radiofrequency imaging uses the differences in electron density (dielectric constant) of the various tissues to directly produce a density map without recourse to the resonance phenomenon. The process of image formation is a special form of inverse scattering analysis that was thought mathematically impossible in 1971; at present there are three separate closed-form solutions. The first successful images of biologic structures were determined in 1977 using this technique, and soft-tissue resolution of about 5 mm is already possible in laboratory demonstration equipment. Again, there is no theoretical limit, but development will be expensive, time-consuming, and probably not very financially rewarding for some years.

APPENDIX 3

SELECTED BIBLIOGRAPHY

Bibliography

Arena, V.: *Ionizing Radiation and Life*. St. Louis: C. V. Mosby, 1971.

Bacq, A.: *Fundamentals of Radiology*. Woburn, Mass.: Butterworth, 1974.

Bushong, S. C.: *Radiologic Science for Technologists*. St. Louis: C. V. Mosby, 1975.

Cheris, D. N., Cheris, B. H.: *Basic Physics and Principles of Diagnostic Radiology*. Chicago: Yearbook Medical Publishers, 1964.

Christensen, E. E., Curry, T. S., Dowdey, J. E.: *An Introduction to the Physics of Diagnostic Radiology*. 2nd Edition. Philadelphia: Lea & Febiger, 1978.

Claus, W. D. (ed.): *Radiation Biology and Medicine, United States Atomic Energy Commission*. Reading, Mass.: Addison-Wesley, 1958.

Daniel, J.: The x-rays. *Science* 3(67):562–563, 1896.

Eastman Kodak: *X-Rays in Dentistry*. Rochester, NY, 1964.

Fuchs, A. W.: *Principles of Radiographic Exposure and Processing*. 2nd Edition. Springfield, Ill.: Charles C Thomas, 1969.

Glasser, O., Taylor, L. S., Quimby, E. H., Weatherwax, J. L., Morgan, R. H.: *Physical Foundations of Radiology*. 3rd Edition. New York: Harper & Row, Hoeber Medical Division, 1965.

Glenner, R. A.: 80 years of dental radiology. *Oral Health* 66(7):10–21, 1976.

Goodwin, P. N., Quimby, E. H., Morgan, R. H.: *Physical Foundations of Radiology*. 4th Edition. New York: Harper & Row, 1970.

Hanawalt, P. C., Cooper, P. K., Ganeson, A. K., Smith, C. A.: *Ann Rev Biochem* 48:783–836, 1979.

Johns, H. E., Cunningham, J. R.: *The Physics of Radiology*. 3rd Edition. Springfield, Ill.: Charles C Thomas, 1974.

Langland, O. E., Sippy, F. H.: *Textbook of Dental Radiology*. Revised 1st Edition. Springfield, Ill.: Charles C Thomas, 1975.

Manson-Hing, L. R.: *Fundamentals of Dental Radiology*. Philadelphia: Lea & Febiger, 1979.

Manson-Hing, L. R.: *Panoramic Dental Radiography*. Springfield, Ill.: Charles C Thomas, 1976.

National Council on Radiation Protection and Measurements Report No. 25, March, 1970.

National Council on Radiation Protection and Measurements Report No. 39, Second Printing June, 1974.

National Council on Radiation Protection and Measurements Report No. 43, January, 1975.

Pizzarello, D. J., Witcofski, R. L.: *Basic Radiation Biology*. 2nd Edition. Philadelphia: Lea & Febiger, 1975.

Reid, J. A., Ruprecht, A.: *Fundamentals of Oral Radiology*. London: Scholar House Publishing, 1976.

Reid, J. A., Ruprecht, A., Stoneman, D. W.: *Practical Radiation Physics*. Saskatoon: University Saskatchewan Press, 1977.

Revel, M., Grones, Y.: Post-transcriptional and translational controls of gene expression in eukaryotes. *Ann Rev Biochem* 47:1079–1126, 1978.

Selman, J.: *The Fundamentals of X-Ray and Radium Physics*. 4th Edition. Springfield, Ill.: Charles C Thomas, 1965.

White, S. C., Blaschke, D. D., Hadley, J. N., Mourshed, F., Sammartino, F. J., Thunthy, K. K.: *Glossary of Dental Radiology*. 2nd Edition. American Academy of Dental Radiology, 1978.

Wuehrmann, A. H., Manson-Hing, L. R.: *Dental Radiology*. 4th Edition. St. Louis: C. V. Mosby, 1977.

INDEX

Note: Page numbers in *italics* indicate illustrations. Page numbers followed by (t) indicate tables. Page numbers followed by (q) indicate sample examination questions.

A (mass number), definition of, 3
Absorption, differential, by tissue(s), 70q, 173q
  photoelectric, 39q
Accelerating agent(s), in film processing, 108t
Acidifier(s) in film processing, 108t
Activated water, definition of, 222
Added filtration, 42
Air-ionization dosimetry, 53q
Alpha particle, of radiation, 24
Aluminum, for filtration, 42, *43,* 46q
Aluminum equivalent(s), of total filtration during primary radiation, 160t
Anatomic accuracy, improving, 61–62, *62*
  with paralleling technique, 74–75q, *74,* 86q, 87q
  with projection technique(s), 61–62, *62*
Angulation, vertical, in buccal-object rule, 78–79, *79,* 80q, *81*
Annihilation reaction, 35
Anode, 10–11, *10, 14,* 19q, 21q
  in x-ray production, 17q
  properties of, 18q
  rotating, 11
  stationary, 11
Anode-film distance, with paralleling technique, 87q
Atom, definition of, 2, 8q
  neutrality of, 2, 7q
  structure of, 2–6, *3–4*
Atomic number (Z), definition of, 3
Automatic film processing, 122–129. See also *Automatic processor.*
  vs. manual processing, 130q
Automatic processor, jamming of, 131q
  maintenance of, 127–129, *128*
  parts of, 122–125, *123, 124,* 125–126t
  solutions in, 126–127
  vs. manual processor, 130q

utomatic temperature control, in darkroom, 120
Autotransformer, *12,* 13

BA (bisecting-angle) technique, *61, 62,* 73q, 84–85, *84*
Background radiation, natural, dose rate from, 151q
Base damage, to DNA, 138–139, *138,* 157q
  to RNA, 138–139
Benson line-focus principle, 66q, *66q*
Bergonie-Tribondeau law, 157
Beta particle, of radiation, 24
Binding energy, 26
  of electron, 7q
Biologic damage, 135–144, 150q
  from Compton effect, 135–136
  from free radical formation, 150q, *150*
  from high-speed electron, 136
  from photoelectric effect, 135–136
  indirect effects vs. direct effects of, 138
  latent period of, 151q
  LET and, 136, *136*
  mechanism of, 155–156q
  repairable, 157q
  theory of, 150q
  to DNA, 138–139, *138,* 157q
  to RNA, 138–139
  to tissue(s), 153q, 155q
Biologic effect(s), of delta ray, 137, *137*
Biologic response, to radiation, 151q
Biologic target(s), of radiation, 137
Bisecting-angle (BA) technique, *61, 62,* 84–85, *84.* See also *Projection technique(s).*
  bite-block(s) used with, 84
  distortion and, 73q, 74q
  foreshortening in, 73q, 74q, 87q

233

Film (*Continued*)
    drying problems of, 125t
    emulsion, for, composition of, 103q, 105q
    extraoral, 95–97, *95,* 101q
      and intensifying screen, 103q
    grain size of, in definition, 58
    handling of, 174q
      errors in, 121, 121t, 122
    herringbone pattern on, 93, 98q, 112q
    Hurter & Driffield curve of, 100q
    intraoral, 91–95, 101q, 104q
      grain of, 92
      sizes of, *94,* 95
      speed of, 92
    occlusal, 101q, 104q. See also *Intraoral film.*
    overdevelopment of, 114q
    processing of. See *Film processing.*
    sensitivity of. See *Film, speed of.*
    speed of, 104q
      and image quality, 100q
      radiation dose with, 99q, 100q, 101q
    type(s) of, 64
    unexposed, 104q
Film badge, as record of x-ray exposure, 52, 54q
Film badge dosimetry, 165q
Film cassette. See *Film packet.*
Film fog, 120
    cause of, 102q, 114q, 116q. See also *Chemical fog.*
    contrast and, 72q
    density and, 72q
    extraoral film and, 96
    factors contributing to, 130q
    from unsafe safelight, 131q
Film gelatin, in developing solution, 116q
Film packet, extraoral, 96–97
    intraoral, 92–95, *92, 93, 94,* 102q
    periapical radiographic, 102q
Film processing, accelerating agent(s) in, 108t
    acidifier(s) in, 108t
    automatic, 122–129. See also *Automatic processor.*
      vs. manual, 130q
    clearing agent(s) in, 108t
    developing solution(s) in, 108t, 113q, 115q
    errors in, 121t, 122
    fixing solution(s) in, 108t, 115q
    hardening agent(s) in, 108t, 118q
    manual, optimum temperature for, 115q
    preservative agent(s) in, 108t
    problems of, 125–126t
    processing solution(s) in, 108t
    reducing agent(s) in, 108t
    restraining agent(s) in, 108t
    solvent agent(s) in, 108t
    surface marks in, 125t
    time-temperature, 110–111, 110t, 113q, 115q
Filter, 223
    darkroom, 120, 120t
    material for, 42, *43,* 46q
    safelight, for developing screen films, 130q
Filtration, added, 42
    inherent, 42
    material for, 42, *43,* 46q
    of long-wavelength photons, 46q

Filtration (*Continued*)
    of long-wavelength x ray(s), 160–161
    of photon(s), 46q
    of x-ray beam, 42, *43*
    purpose of, 160–161
    reducing scattered radiation fog by, 47q
    small focal spot and, 68–69q
    total, 42, 46q
Fitzgerald, F. G., 171, 174q
Fixed image, 108, *109*
Fixing solution(s) in film processing, 108t, 115q
    component(s) of, 117q
    replenishing of, 126–127
    temperature of, 110–111, 110t
Fixing time, 110–111, 110t, 114q, 115q
Focal spot (FS), *14, 15,* 67q, *68*q
    image projection and, 57
    leakage radiation and, 22q
    size of, 68q
      Benson line-focus principle and, 66q, *66*q
      definition and, 58, 63, 67q
      detail and, 63
      filtration and, 68–69q
      penumbra and, 68–69q
Focal spot-film distance (FFD),
    definition and, 69q
    exposure time and, 90q
    in paralleling technique, 86q
    magnification and, 69q
Focal spot–object distance, exposure time and, 90q
Focus-film distance, and penumbra, 64
Fog on x-ray film. See *Film fog.*
Foreshortening, 60–61, *61*
    in bisecting-angle technique, 73q, 74q, 87q
Free radical formation, biologic damage from, 150q, *150*q
FS (focal spot), *14, 15,* 67q, 68q

General radiation, 28q
Genetic damage, from radiation, 134, 139, 140–143
Genetic mutation, definition of, 223
Geometric factor(s), in image quality, 55–65
Geometric unsharpness. See *Penumbra.*
Glaucoma, from ionizing radiation, 144
Gonad(s), effects of radiation on, 140–143, 141t
    protection of, in dental radiography, 161
    radiosensitivity of, 142, 149q
Gray (Gy), definition of, 156q
Grid(s), definition of, 223
    use of, in radiography, 96, 99q
      patient exposure and, 99q
Gy (Gray), definition of, 156q

Half-value layer (HVL), 36, 47q
    measurement of, 50–52
Hardening agent(s), in film processing, 108t, 118q
Heat, and bremsstrahlung radiation, *26*
    dissipation of, during x-ray production, 21q

Herringbone pattern, on film, 93, 98q, 112q
Heterogeneous x-ray beam, 42
High-speed electron, biologic damage from, 136
  energy loss of, 155q
  LET of, 136, *136*
High-voltage circuit, in step-up transformer, 12
Hurter & Driffield curve, of film, 100q
HVL (half-value layer), 36, 47q
Hydrogen, atomic structure of, *3*

Image, cone-cutting on, 98q
  contrast of, 63, 71q, 116q
  definition of, 56, 58–59, *58, 59.* See also *Sharpness.*
  density of, 63
  detail in, 63–64
  dimensional distortion of, 56–57, *56,* 60–61, *61*
  fixed, 108, *109*
  latent, 64–65, 99q, 108, *109,* 117q
  magnification of, 56–57, *56*
  overlapping of, 60–61, *61,* 66q
  partial, 98q
  penumbra of, 57
  processed, 108
  projection principles of, 57–58, 66q
  quality of, 55–65
    film speed and, 100q
  unfixed, 108, *109*
  unsharpness of, 55–57, *56*
Image processing, automatic, 122–129
  chemistry of, 107–111, 108t, 110t, 112q, 117q
  defective, cause of, 116q
  errors in, 121t, 122
  manual, 115q, 130q
  problems of, 125–126t
  solutions in, 112q
Image projection, focal spot and, 57
Image shift, in buccal-object rule, 82q
Incident photon, 35
  ionization and, 5, *5*
Incident viewing light, and radiographic density, 131q
Incoherent scatter, definition of, 224
Inherent filtration, 42
Input coil, of transformer, 12–13, *12*
Intensifying screen(s), 98q, 103q
  comparison of speeds of, 98q
  extraoral, 95–97, *95,* 99q
    radiation dose with, 99q
  fast-speed, 98q
  intraoral, 95
  screen film and, 102q
  slow-speed, 98q
  use of with extraoral film, 103q
Intraoral film, 91–95, 101q, 104q
  grain of, 92
  sizes of, *94,* 95
  speed of, 92
Intraoral film packet, 92–95, *92, 93, 94,* 102q
  use of lead in, 102q
Intraoral intensifying screen(s), 95

Intraoral projection technique(s), 84–85, *84, 85*
Inverse square law, 36, 85
  formula for, 88q, 89
Ion, definition of, 222
Ion pair, definition of, 222
Ionization, 37q
  definition of, 222
  incident photon and, 5, *5*
  of matter, 4–5, *5,* 7q
  x rays and, 7q
Ionizing radiation, 37q. See also *Radiation.*
Iron, in x-ray tube, 12
Isobar(s), definition of, 6
Isotope(s), definition of, 5, *6*

Kells, C. E., 170, 173q
Kiloelectron volt (keV), 135
Kilovoltage (kV), 13, 14, 22q
  and penetrative quality of radiation, 17q, 19q
  contrast and, 63, 70q, 72q
  definition and, 69q
  electron velocity and, 22q
  radiation produced by, 18q, 20q, 29q
Kilovoltage peak (kVp), 13, 14, 18q, 20q
  effect of, on radiograph, 20q
  long-scale contrast and, 71q
Kinetic energy, definition of, 223
kV (kilovoltage), 13, 14
kVp (kilovoltage peak), 13, 14, 18q, 20q
  density and, 70q, 71q, 72q
  long-scale contrast and, 71q
  photon wavelength and, 18q
  short-scale contrast and, 13

Latent effect of radiation, leukemia as, 151q
Latent image, 64–65, 99q, 108, *109,* 117q
LD$_{50}$ (lethal dose), of radiation, 154q
Lead, as protection for dental personnel, 163
  in collimator, 44, 46q
  in intraoral film packet, 102q
  in x-ray machine, 47q
  to reduce scattered radiation fog, 47q
Leaded apron, 140, 161, 165q
Leakage radiation, 22q, 160
LET (linear energy transfer), and biologic damage, 136, *136*
  Bragg peak of, 136, *136*
  definition of, 224
  low, definition of, 224
  of high-speed electron, 136, *136*
Lethal dose (LD$_{50}$), of radiation, 154q
Leukemia, as latent effect of radiation, 151q
  from occupational radiation exposure, 153q
Linear energy transfer (LET), and biologic damage, 136, *136*
  Bragg peak of, 136, *136*
  definition of, 224
  low, definition of, 224
  of high-speed electron, biologic damage from, 136, *136*

237

Oral cavity, effect of therapeutic radiation on, 143–144
Organogenesis, radiation-induced anomalies in, 155q
Orthopantomograph, 172
Osteoradionecrosis, from occupational radiation exposure, 153q
  in jaws, 143
Output coil, of transformer, 12–13, *12*, 20q
Overdevelopment of film, 114q
Overexposure, to radiation, observable reaction to, 151–152q
Overlapping of radiographic image, 60–61, *61,* 66q
Oxygen, atomic structure of, *3*

P technique, 61, *62, 73*q, 74q, 84–85, *85*
Paatero, Y. V., 172, 174q
Pair production, 34–35, *35*
Panoramic radiography, 97, 174q
Pantomography, radiation dose during, 148t
Paralleling (P) technique, *61, 62, 73*q, 74q, 84–85, *85*
  advantages of, 85, 86q
  anatomic accuracy with, 74–75q, *74,* 86q, 87q
  angle in, 88q
  anode-film distance with, 87q
  collimator with, 84, 85
  cone-positioning device with, 84, 85
  developing time with, 86q
  extension cone as adjunct to, 86q
  extension long-cone, 171
  focal spot–film distance in, 86q
  long cone with, 74–75q, *74,* 86q, 87q. See also *Long-cone technique.*
  modified (MP), *73*q, 74q
  object-film distance with, 87q
  target-film distance with, 87q
Partial image, 98q
Particle(s) of radiation, 24
Particulate radiation, 24, 31q
Patient, dental, radiation and, 135–144, 165q
  protection of, 161–163
  use of grids and, 99q
Peak kilovoltage. See *Kilovoltage peak.*
Penumbra, *56,* 57, 64
  and definition, 58–59, *58, 59*
  calculating zone of, 59
  decreasing size of, 58–59, *58, 59*
  definition and, 58–59, *58, 59*
  definition of, 225
  focus-film distance and, 64
  object-film distance and, 64
  short-cone technique and, *72*q, *73*q
  small focal spot and, 68–69q
  source-object distance and, 58–59, *58, 59*
  unsharpness of, 64
Periapical radiograph(s), 104q. See also *Intraoral film.*
Personnel monitoring, for radiation protection, 163, 164q. See also *Dosimetry.*
Photoelectric absorption, 39q
  ionization and, 37q

Photoelectric collision, 35
Photoelectric effect, 34, *35,* 37, *37*q, 38q, 39q
  biologic damage from, 135–136
Photoelectron, 35
Photon(s), definition of, 224
  energy range of, in dentistry, 135
  filtration of, 46q
  incident, 35
    and ionization, 5, *5*
  long-wavelength, filtration of, 46q
  of electromagnetic energy, 24
  production of, energy transformation in, 17q
  scattered, 34, *35*
  wavelength of, and kilovoltage peak, 18q
Photon energy range, of x-ray beam, in dentistry, 135
Photonuclear disintegration, 39q
Pocket dosimetry, 50–52, *51,* 53q, 54q
Pointed cone(s), scattered radiation with, 84
Polychromatic x-ray beam, 42
Positron, 35, *35*
  definition of, 223
Pregnancy, and dental radiography, 164q
Preservative agent(s), in film processing, 108t
Primary coil, of transformer, 12–13, *12*
Primary radiation, 30q, 160
Primary x-ray beam, 42
Processed image, 108
Processing solution(s), in film processing, 108t
Projection, rules of, 57–58, 66q
Projection technique(s), anatomic accuracy in, 61–62, *62*
  bisecting-angle, *61, 62, 73*q, 74q, 84–85, *84*
  bite-wing, 88q, 93
  definition with, 58–59, *58, 59*
  dimensional distortion in, 60–61, *61*
  extension long-cone paralleling, 171
  intraoral, 84–85, *84, 85*
  long cone, 72q, *73*q, 86q. See also *Paralleling technique.*
  long-cone paralleling, development of, 171, 174q
  magnification in, 59–60, *60*
  maxillary occlusal, 81q
  modified paralleling, *73*q, 74q
  objectives of, 58–62
  paralleling, *61, 62, 73*q, 74q, 84–85, *85*
  rectangular collimation, 171
  right-angle, 82q
  short-cone, *61,* 72q, *73*q, 74–75q, *74*q. See also *Bisecting-angle technique.*
Proton(s), definition of, 2, *2,* 223
  of particulate radiation, 24

QF (quality factor), 50
  rem and, 53q
Quality assurance program, in dental office, 162
Quality factor (QF), 50
  rem and, 53q
Quantum, definition of, 224
Quantum mottle, 224

239

R (roentgen unit), 50
Rad (radiation absorbed dose), 50, 54q
  definition of, 50, 222
  formula for, 223
Radiant energy, definition of, 224
Radiation, absorption of, by bone, 149q
    by film, 100q
  alpha particle of, 24
  and dental patients, 135–144
  and use of leaded apron, 140
  average entrance skin dose of, 147t
  background, natural, dose rate from, 151q
  beta particle of, 24
  biologic damage from, in dentistry,
    135–144. See also *Biologic damage.*
  biologic effects of, 133–148
  biologic response to, 151q
  biologic targets of, 137
  bone marrow dose of, 148t
  Bremsstrahlung, 25, *26,* 27, 37q
    definition of, 224
  cell sensitivity to, 149q, 153q, 157
    factors in, 150q
  characteristic, 26–27, *26,* 40q
  chromosomal aberrations caused by, 142
  dissipation of heat during production of,
    21q
  doubling dose of, 156q
  effect(s) of, non-dose-related, 154q
    on fetal tissue, 140
    on function of cells, 139
    on organogenesis, 155q
  electromagnetic, 24–27, *25,* 28q
    definition of, 225
  energy of, 24–27
  erythema from, 139–140, 154–155q
  exit dose of, 44, *45*
  from high kilovoltage, 18q, 20q, 29q
  general, 28q
  genetic damage from, 134, 139, 140–143
  glaucoma from, 144
  gonadal effects of, 140–143, 141t
  hazards of, 170–171
    to dental personnel, 166–167q
  interaction with water of, 137–138
  leakage of, 22q, 160
  lethal dose (LD$_{50}$) of, 154q
  leukemia from, 151q
  maximum permissible dose (MPD) of,
    145–146, 147t, 150q, 154q
  measurement(s) of, 49–52, *51,* 52t
  mid-lethal dose of, clinical symptoms of,
    155q
  nature of, x-rays and, 23–27
  nonparticulate, 32q
  occupational exposure to. See *Dental
    personnel, radiation exposure of.*
  oral mucositis from, 143
  overexposure to, observable reaction to,
    151–152q
  particulate, 24, 31q
  penetrative quality of, 17q
  primary, 30q, 160
  properties of, magnification and, 67q
  protection from, 159–163, 160t
    and aluminum equivalents, 160, 160t
    and cone diameter, 160

Radiation, protection from (*Continued*)
    collimator as, 165q
    of patient, 161–163
    of thyroid, 161
    personnel monitoring for, 163, 164q
  quantity of, and high kilovoltage, 18q, 20q,
    29q
    and milliamperage, 20q
  scattered, 34, 160
    biologic damage from, 135
    definition of, 224
    reduction of, 47q
    with pointed cone(s), 84
  secondary, 30q, 160, 166q. See also
    Radiation, scattered.
    as hazard to dental personnel, 165q
    control of, 167q
    definition of, 225
  somatic effects of, 134
  specific-region, 152q
  therapeutic, effect(s) of, on oral cavity,
    143–144
    purpose of, 152q
    tissue destruction in, 152q
    threshold dose of, 152q
  tissue susceptibility to, 149q
  to cervical spine, in dental radiography,
    148t
  unnecessary, 44
  "white." See *Radiation, bremsstrahlung.*
  whole-body, 134–135, 152q
Radiation absorbed dose (rad), 50, 54q
Radiation caries, 143
Radiation dose, during cephalometry, 147t
  during pantomography, 148t
  film speed and, 99q, 100q, 101q
  from dental radiography, 141t
  to patient, reduction of, 165q
  to skin, in diagnostic radiography, 147t
  with Clark's rule, 80q
  with extraoral intensifying screen, 99q
Radiation mucositis, in oral cavity, 143
Radiation output, source-film distance and,
    90q
Radiation safety. See *Radiation, protection
    from.*
Radiatized film, 64
Radical, free, formation of, biologic damage
    from, 150q, *150*
Radiobiology, 133–148
Radiograph, density of, and incident viewing
    light, 131q
    reducing, 117q
  effect of kVp on, 20q
  first intraoral, 170
  periapical, 104q. See also *Intraoral film.*
  resolution on, 65
  viewing of, 129
Radiographic burnout, definition of, 225
Radiographic image. See *Image.*
Radiography, dental, bone marrow dose in,
    148t
  patient protection in, 161–163
  pregnancy and, 164q
  radiation dose, during, 141t
  to cervical spine, 148t
  diagnostic, 147t

242